Second Opinion's

Practical Guide to Home Remedies

Second Opinion's

Practical Guide to Home Remedies

564 safe, all-natural ways to prevent and cure scores of common illnesses, problems and complaints

by Steven E. Kroening
Managing Editor, *Second Opinion*

Foreward by William Campbell Douglass, MD

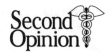

Second Opinion Publishing
Atlanta, Georgia

Cover illustration by Elizabeth Bame

ISBN 1-885236-10-7

Library of Congress Catalog Card Number
95-92924

Second Opinion Publishing also publishes Dr. William Campbell Douglass' monthly "contrary opinion" medical newsletter, *Second Opinion*. To subscribe or obtain a free catalog describing all Second Opinion products, please call or write:

Soundview Publications, Inc.
P.O. Box 467939
Atlanta, Georgia 31146-7939
800-728-2288 or 770-399-5617

Table of Contents

Dedication

This book is dedicated to my mom, Eva Kroening, who taught me to not only strive for a goal, but to keep going until I've reached it.

Acknowledgements

There were several people who made this book what it is today. First, I'd like to say "thank you" to God, who is the Great Healer and Provider. In spite of our sin against Him, he still gives us provision: "Their fruit will serve for food and their leaves for healing." (Ezekiel 47:12)

I would also like to thank my new wife, Beth, for her patients with my "crazy ideas." And to my parents and brothers for their love and encouragement through the years.

Next, this book never would have happened were it not for my publishers and bosses, Chip and Garret Wood, who have provided me with a wonderful opportunity. For this I will be forever grateful. You've put together a great staff, who I would also like to thank for their continued encouragement.

And finally, a special word of appreciation is extended to all of you who wrote in with your contributions. May they encourage the healing of many others.

Foreword

Now I'm not one to claim that nutritional supplements or carrot juice can cure all that ails you. And, like you, I'm fed up with those idiotic claims you find in the tabloid press: "Lose Weight Overnight While You Sleep," "Miracle Vitamin Cream Erases Wrinkles Instantly," or "Special Men's Supplement Gives You the Spark of Youth."

Those who make such unrealistic claims do more harm than good and they turn most people off to the real value of supplements. Americans are so bombarded with these fabrications that when vitamins, minerals, and "health foods" are found to have real value, their value may be ignored. That's because the press has conditioned them to believe these things to be useless in the treatment and prevention of disease.

So people don't know what to believe: their doctor isn't qualified in this field, the FDA is a corrupt and self-serving bureaucracy, and the health-oriented portion of the press often exaggerates the benefits of nutrients — just as the bureaucrats in the FDA say it does.

But the FDA's answer is the RDA (recommended daily allowance), which began 40 years ago — and hasn't changed much since. Back in those days, people were worried about rickets and scurvy, not about helping themselves maintain optimum health in the face of processed foods, processed water, and unprocessed contaminated air. The RDA gives the *minimum* amount of a vitamin or mineral needed to maintain *minimum* health. There's nothing optimum about these allowances, and they ignore all of the research that's been done over the last four decades — research that shows the healing power and preventive abilities of some foods, herbs, and nutritional supplements. So the FDA's not much help.

That's where *At-Home Remedies* comes in. Some of the remedies you'll read in this book are very recent discoveries. But many others are generations old. Our forefathers didn't know that carrots contain beta carotene, but they knew carrots were good for you, particularly if you were having a vision problem. My great-grandmother used to say, "Don't tell the patient your grandma is going to cure them. Just tell them, with God's help, she will help you get better."

This book contains the wisdom of some of the best alternative health doctors and specialists in the world. They know what works and what doesn't from both conventional and alternative medicine. What they have to say may not cure everything that ails you, but with God's help, it could help you get better.

William Campbell Douglass, MD
October 1996

Introduction

My great-grandfather started driving cattle from Texas to Kansas when he was eleven years old. Granddad made his living as an itinerant farm worker during the dust-bowl days of the Great Depression. Then there was my mother, who was the first child from her family born in a house (if you could call it that) — the first eight children were born in a tent.

With such a lifestyle, doctors were not a luxury my ancestors could afford very often. Instead, they took care of themselves. How well? Granddad lived into his 80s, Granny into her 90s. They ate bacon and eggs almost every morning, straight from their own hogs and chickens, and didn't worry a dime about their cholesterol count. I don't think they ever heard of such a thing.

That's the kind of family I was born into. I remember staying home from school with any assortment of illnesses when I was a child, thinking I needed to go to the doctor. Mom knew better. It wasn't that she didn't like the doctor, she just knew when it was time to go. That's how I first got started with home remedies. I didn't pay much attention back then, but the attitude of taking responsibility for my own health was well ingrained.

All too often, home remedies are used as a last ditch effort by a patient who has "tried everything else" that conventional medicine has to offer. That's the wrong way to do it. We should try everything we can at home first. If it doesn't work, *then* we should go to the doctor. This simple change in attitude could save you a bundle on doctor's bills. It could also improve your health. (Obviously, certain conditions require immediate medical attention — if it's serious and getting worse fast, do yourself a favor and call the doc.)

What you'll find in this book is the first step toward better health. Treating yourself will inspire great confidence and promote enduring well-being. Of course, for those of you who have already been to the doctor, feel free to use it as a last resort or even a second opinion. You'll be glad you did.

Steven E. Kroening
October 1996

Section 1

Pain

Chapter 1

Stop the Pain

Tom was in pain. "He no longer took an interest in war, nor even in piracy. The charm of life was gone; there was nothing but dreariness left. He put his hoop away, and his bat; there was no joy in them any more."

Young Mr. Sawyer's ailment may have been only love pains, but it was still serious enough to put a damper on life. That's the way pain is. No matter what form it comes in, it's no laughing matter. And the quicker you can get rid of it, the happier you'll be.

When Tom Sawyer's aunt became concerned about Tom's pain she immediately "began to try all manner of remedies on him." She deluged him with cold water, gave him "hot baths, sitz baths, shower baths, and plunges," but nothing seemed to work. Does the situation sound familiar?

If you're experiencing a headache, backache, or any other type of pain, you'll probably try anything just to be free from the agony. Unfortunately, pain is a very personal problem and usually requires a personal method of dealing with it. Some treatments for specific ailments work for everybody across the board, but others work for only a few individuals here and there.

The drug industry has always been swift to provide pain sufferers with a "quick fix" solution to their problem. Sometimes they work, sometimes they don't. But many, if not most of them, have some sort of side effect if they're used over an extended period of time.

Aspirin, for instance, is the most popular pain reliever on the market. Americans consume 15 tons of aspirin every day (that's about 19 billion tablets per year) and the Aspirin Foundation boasts that the chemical "probably has been taken, at one time or another, by almost every human being on earth." But according to a Mayo Clinic report, aspirin can cause chronic duodenal ulcers and bleeding from the duodenum. Dr. William Campbell Douglass, author of *Dangerous (Legal) Drugs*, says, "Every time you take an aspirin you bleed a little into your gut. A microscope will show every time that the bowel movement of someone on daily aspirin contains blood."

You're trying to kill your pain, not add another source of it. You want safe, easy-to-administer solutions to your health problems and a little bit of help can go a long way. You need to find remedies that you can use to alleviate the pain, and ***Second Opinion's Practical Guide to Home Remedies*** has them.

So beginning with headaches, we're going to follow Tom Sawyer's steps by taking matters into our own hands and start thinking "over various plans for relief."

Chapter 2

Headaches

Everybody has suffered from the pain of a throbbing headache at some point in their life. So common is the problem, in fact, that more than 45 million Americans suffer from headaches time and time again. And of those, 16 to 18 million suffer from migraines.

The search for a remedy has become a multibillion dollar industry. But the difficulty doesn't come in finding a treatment for a headache — it's finding a remedy that actually works, without side effects.

If you spend $50 for a visit to your doctor, he's probably not going to tell you anything different than what you would find in most home remedy books. In fact, by doing a little homework you would probably save time and money and know more about your problem. But even many of the home remedy books are short on effective answers for that stubborn headache.

The standard answers for headaches will oftentimes work. They include: relax, get some exercise, get some sleep, breathe deeply, watch your caffeine intake, don't chew gum, go easy on the salt, and don't smoke. All of those are valid recommendations and should be your starting point, especially for normal tension headaches.

But if you've tried all the usual remedies and find that they don't work, it's time to do some logical thinking.

Pain: The Body's Warning Sign

Anytime you experience a pain sensation, your body is sending you a warning signal that something is wrong. Many of the remedies we use on a daily basis are directed at stopping the pain, not correcting the problem. Is there a difference? Yes! Modern medicine has become very efficient at dulling the body's nervous system to a point where no pain can be felt. But just because the pain is gone doesn't mean you're out of danger. The aching part of your body can send the brain all the messages it wants. But if the nerves won't carry the message, the brain doesn't know that it needs to react.

Dr. H.C.A. Vogel, author of *The Nature Doctor*, makes a strong statement that should be heeded by all chronic headache sufferers in their search for a cure. He says: "Let me point out that a headache *per se* is never an illness, only a symptom pointing to an illness that is causing it." Therefore, taking a painkiller is often an inappropriate action and may cause more problems by giving you a false sense of safety.

When you've experienced pain in the past, how many times were you thankful your body warned you that something needed to be fixed? Even more important, will you take the time to find out what is causing the pain? Most of us wouldn't. But when chronic headaches, or any chronic pain for that matter, plagues us, we should investigate. If you want to rid yourself of constant headache pain, it is fundamentally important to find and treat the cause. Otherwise, the pain will return, again and again.

Dr. Vogel says, "Merely alleviating pain, the symptom, will be of no service to the body. People who habitually swallow analgesics little realize that their constant headaches may well be due to persistent constipation. Who would think that the toxins remaining in the bowels could be the cause of such headaches?...

"Putrefactive processes develop gases which enter the liver through the portal vein and, from there, find their way into the bloodstream. Headaches frequently result because the nerve and brain cells are affected by the poisons circulating in the blood." If you think constipation is the cause of your headache, try drinking some carrot juice. (If that doesn't work, see page 179.)

Other Causes

In addition to intestinal disturbances, the Bircher-Benner Headache Clinic in Zurich, Switzerland says that

---

Headaches from Food Preservatives

"I am writing you concerning a home discovery of a medical problem. It is regarding severe headaches caused by common food preservatives. These occur 18 to 24 hours after ingestion of the preservatives BHA or BHT, and rather sooner after ingestion of Sodium Benzoate or Potassium Sorbate. I have several others on a suspect list, but I try to avoid them all! I am not generally subject to allergies." — *L.A., Maryland*

headaches can be caused by metabolic overload, arteriosclerosis, heart ailments, disorders of the liver or kidney, abdominal troubles and diseases, ruptured or slipped discs, high or low blood pressure, diseases of the blood, and nephritis. Other times a headache might be from a narrowed space in the skull, mental illness, heat and sunstroke, sinus congestion, infectious disease, tuberculosis, eye strain, neuralgia, shingles, and allergies. Remember that if your headache is due to one of these, the disorder must be healed before the headache will be alleviated.

In addition to these, Dr. Vogel said: "Headaches can also be caused by insufficient blood supply to the brain. In this case we recommend ... Ginkgo biloba, also known as maidenhair tree. The leaves of this tree contain active properties that can do wonders for the cerebral blood supply.

"Physical therapy should not be forgotten either. Relief is often obtained from warm showers directed on the nape of the neck and the spine, as well as massaging with Toxeucal Massage Oil. If the headaches stem from an upset digestive system, warm showers directed on the stomach are the answer to alleviating the pain."

Contraction vs. Expansion

Annemarie Colbin, author of *Food and Healing*, gives a much easier way to classify simple headaches. She says that most headaches are "caused by (a) expansion of the blood vessels in the head; or (b) tension or strain of the muscles in the neck, scalp, or face." The first group describes headaches that fall into the vascular (expansion) category, while the headaches in the second group are classified as tension headaches (contraction). Colbin also has "side categories for 'liver' headaches, caffeine-withdrawal headaches, and others."

Expansion headaches are usually caused by drinking too much liquid of any kind or eating too much ice cream or other cold and highly sugared food. These are best treated by eating some Gomasio, Umeboshi plums, or brine-cured olives. Gomasio is made by grinding "1 cup roasted sesame seeds, until half crushed, in a mortar, preferably the Japanese kind known as a suribachi, which has grooves. Add 2 teaspoons sea salt; then grind the salt well into the seeds." Umeboshi plums are also called plums pickled in brine and can be found in Japanese and health food stores. You can expect these remedies to work in two to 15 minutes.

Contraction headaches, on the other hand, are the result of too much tension, heat, meats and salty foods, mental concentration, or a lack of food and/or fluids. The best remedies for these include apple or apricot juice and cold unsweetened applesauce or other cooked fruit. The headache should be gone in five minutes to 24 hours.

Liver headaches, or migraines, are similar to contraction headaches, only stronger, more painful, and harder to ease. According to Colbin, "They arise two, four, even eight hours after the unbalancing food has been consumed and therefore are rarely linked to it. Usually, they are the result of consuming fatty foods on an empty stomach, including fried eggs or cheese for breakfast, fried tofu or tempeh, salads with oily dressings, avocados, and tempura."

The remedies for a migraine are the same as listed above for the contraction headache, but you can also try lemon tea and a five-phase drink. (Mix 1 cup lemon tea

Help for Cluster Headache Sufferers

"My cluster headaches began in 1948 at age 19. They were first accurately diagnosed as histamine cephalalgia, confirmed by injecting a bit of histamine into the arm. This reproduced the headache symptoms in every detail.... The origin of the histamine remained a mystery until it finally proved to be due to sensitivity/allergy to several foods such as apricots (a favorite on morning toast) and oats (cereal, bread, cookies, etc.). Opening a jar or package with one of these and eating some almost every day would soon lead to headaches. Up to three a day, for however long one of these foods was eaten. The pain is one-sided, about like that of a bad toothache, lasts up to two or three hours, then fades, leaving one numb and washed out. It can come at any time, so it can be very wearing on the sufferer and those who live in the same house.

"Dr. Arthur Coca, author of *The Pulse Test*, has his readers take their pulse before meals, then three times afterward at half-hour intervals. With one of the more serious problem foods, pulse rates increase above the 'normal' by up to 30 beats per minute, for as long as two hours. No subtlety there. But you have to be a fanatic about keeping records of what is eaten and when, and about reading labels on foods. Eventually, the suspected culprits can be identified, avoided for some days, then eaten to check their effect. One by one, you can learn what must be avoided, or at least kept to tolerable levels of use. With diligence, I am now free of this monster. I am also seriously limited in what I can eat, but it's worth it." — *R.A.B., Oregon*

with 1 tablespoon maple syrup or to taste. Add pinch of cayenne or five drops of Tabasco or 1/2 teaspoon freshly grated ginger. Stir well, drink hot.)

If you are unsure of the type of headache you have, Corbin says to do one of the following to find out:

1. "Make a list of what you've eaten in the past six hours or so and see if it's expansive, contractive, or fatty.

2. "Have a tiny bite of umeboshi plum if you can't figure it out. If you remain the same, or get better, you have an expansive headache. If you get worse, you have a contractive or a liver headache."

A Nutritional Approach

If you read the statistics, most health professionals would probably agree with Ms. Colbin and say that the most common type of headache is due to muscle contraction, also known as the tension headache. So common is this diagnosis, in fact, that one publication estimated that 90 percent of all headaches are tension related.

While this may seem high, this estimation is not uncommon and very little evidence has been shown to refute it. But there are people who do not believe that tension is the number one cause of headaches for most Americans. Dr. Jonathan Wright, one of today's leading figures in nutritional therapy, suggests that spinal problems, allergy or food sensitivities, and blood sugar difficulties are the three main causes of headaches.

In his book, *Guide to Healing with Nutrition*, Dr. Wright says, "If all these causes are properly searched for and treated when found, the number of headaches truly due to tension becomes very small.

"Some headaches diagnosed as migraine can be relieved by removal of refined sugar, processed foods, and by adding more frequent small meals, and other hypoglycemia treatment.... As I've observed many migraine headaches ... partly or completely relieved with hypoglycemia diagnosis and treatment, I think hypoglycemia should be looked for in all headache sufferers, including those said to have migraines."

Most physicians often overlook, or ignore, hypoglycemia and treat migraines as an extreme case of muscle contraction. Dr. Wright says, "In my experience, as well as that of most nutrition-oriented physicians, low blood sugar, or hypoglycemia, is found to be one of the most frequent causes of headaches."

In addition to low blood sugar, Dr. Wright insists that many headaches "appear to be due to food sensitivity, including allergy." Another fact that is ignored by many physicians.

If you've tried everything else and nothing seems to alleviate the pain of chronic headaches, you might try eliminating milk, cheese, eggs, wheat, and coffee from your diet. According to Dr. Wright, a "common cause of headaches — migraine and other types — is food allergy." If, over the course of a week or two, your headaches have gotten better or worse, you know you have a food allergy. This test is not a conclusive means to determine what the allergy is, but it might give you an idea. If the test is positive or if allergies run in your family, you should visit an allergist for more definitive results.

Dehydration

Another major cause of headaches, especially for the elderly and children, that few people recognize is dehydration. Children get dehydrated easily in the summer when they're playing hard and spending a lot of time in the sun. Older adults simply don't drink enough of the right types of liquid. Water, seltzer water, and herb teas should be drunk throughout the day as they contain no caffeine, sugar, or calories. Drinks that contain caffeine and sugar, such as soda and coffee, should be avoided for treating dehydration.

Drinking eight glasses of water a day is the best way to avoid dehydration. But for a little variety, Susan A. Skolnick, author of *The I Feel Awful Cook Book*, says that mixing 1/2 cup seltzer water or club soda, 1/2 cup fruit juice, 1 teaspoon lemon juice, and ice in a glass makes an excellent natural soda to drink when you're dehydrated.

Chapter 3

Backaches

Like headaches, backaches are becoming one of the plagues of the late 20th century. The sedentary lifestyle for most of the American population is a major contributor to the problem. But, ironically, many people suffer back problems from too much or improper exercise.

Dealing with backache is a delicate issue and, in most cases, is not one that should be taken lightly. That doesn't mean that there are not things you can do at home. In fact, there are a number of measures that you should try before you pay a visit to your doctor.

Prevention

The first, of course, is prevention. The following are just some simple guidelines that you should practice on a daily basis.

● Sit up straight. You sit crooked more than you think. If you rest your arm on the window of your car while you drive or lounge on your couch while watching TV, you're throwing your spine off balance on a regular basis.

NAC Helps Prevent Muscle Damage

You have probably heard that vitamins C and E fight the free-radicals in your blood that may contribute to the effects of aging and some diseases. Now there's a new antioxidant on the block that is as effective as C and E, if not more so.

A study recently conducted in Finland found that the antioxidant N-acetylcysteine (NAC) is not only an effective protector from oxidative damage, but may actually eliminate it. This is especially good news for anyone who exercises regularly, as exercise is known to cause free-radicals to form in the body. NAC also dramatically reduces the amount of damage done to the muscles during exercise.

The study found that those who received a placebo had significantly higher levels of oxidized glutathione, one indicator of oxidative damage, after they exercised. While those patients who were given NAC suffered no such increase.

To receive the benefits of NAC you need to take only 200 mg daily. This doesn't sound like a lot, but if you're already taking other antioxidant supplements, like vitamins C and E, it should be more than enough. Evidence indicates that there is a synergistic effect between the supplements. This means for overall health, taking smaller amounts of several different antioxidants is more effective than larger doses of one individual antioxidant.

There is one thing you should know about NAC before you rush out and buy it. NAC contains sulfur so you can imagine what it smells like. If you add this antioxidant to your list of supplements, don't be shocked when you catch a whiff. (*Muscle & Fitness*, 12/94; *Acta Physiologica Scandinavia*, 151:149-154, 1994; *Journal of Applied Physiology*, 76:2570-2577, 1994)

• "Don't slouch!" We've all heard our parents tell us this, but standing properly may involve more than not slouching. When standing for long periods of time, don't switch from one leg to the other. It may feel better on your legs, but it throws your back off balance.

• Use your legs when you lift heavy objects, not your back.

• Avoid sleeping on your stomach, it puts the most strain on your spine. It is best to sleep in a fetal position with a pillow between your legs. Or, if you prefer to sleep on your back, put a small pillow under the hollow of your back.

Acute vs. Chronic Pain

Most back doctors will tell you that there are two types of backache: acute and chronic. Acute pain comes when you're doing something you shouldn't be doing or when you're doing something the wrong way. This form of pain is usually associated with the muscles in the back and can be excruciating for several days.

The most typical treatment for acute pain entails staying off your feet and getting some bed rest. That's definitely the place to start, but that's not all you can do.

Anytime you sprain, strain, or pull a muscle, whether it be in your back or the back of your leg, the same treatments can be used. When an athlete pulls a hamstring or sprains an ankle, the first thing the trainer will do is apply ice for the first 24 hours. This will help keep the swelling down and promote the healing process. The best way to apply ice is to put it in a water bag with some salt. The salt will keep the water from freezing and the bag will conform to the shape of your body.

After the first day of nothing but ice, the trainer will begin an intermittent regimen of heat and ice. Dr. Edward Abraham, author of *Freedom from Back Pain*, says, "Do 30 minutes of ice, then 30 minutes of heat, and keep repeating the cycle." This will exercise the muscle by gently expanding and contracting it and will speed the recovery process. This same treatment can be used very effectively on your back.

Be careful not to apply heat by itself for an extended period of time. While it might feel great, it will increase the swelling and can also make the problem much worse by increasing internal hemorrhaging and causing edema.

Sam Biser, editor of *The Newsletter of Advanced Natural Therapies*, said, "One case was a young fellow of 27 who had strained his back playing tennis. He treated himself for two months with a heating pad. At the end of two months, the pain was spreading to the groin area and down to his thighs. He was a cripple." But after he applied ice, he was able to walk again in a few days.

More Relief for Acute Pain

Another way you can relieve the pain is with a gentle massage. The *Dictionary of the Best Tips and Secrets for Better Health* says to start by locating "the painful points in your back as precisely as possible. Ask a friend to massage these points (pressure can be light or hard depending on your preference, but should not cause more discomfort).

"Then ask the person to massage the same points on the opposite side of your back, pressing much more deeply."

The *Dictionary* also says that applying magnets with bandaids to the painful areas will help soothe the pain in a few minutes. This can be extremely useful for the person who is unwilling or unable to take it easy for a few days.

Other treatments you may want to try include alternating compresses of clay and cabbage leaves or applying a single compress soaked in red pepper tincture. Red pepper is famous for its stimulating and warming properties. Because of this, commercial ointments for soothing muscular and back pain often use red pepper as an ingredient. You can also apply a compress soaked in a decoction of two to four grams of pepper boiled in a litre of water and filtered.

Dr. Vogel recommends the use of a good warming ointment. "It is also beneficial to place some moist, hot hay flowers or camomile, tied in cloth, on the painful area," says Dr. Vogel. These will help to soothe the pain.

If your pain is due to inflammation, Dr. Milton Fried of the Fried Clinic in Atlanta, Georgia recommends that you try some white willow bark. "It is a natural salicylate, the active ingredient that gives aspirin its anti-inflammatory power. Taken after meals, it shouldn't hurt your stomach, and it works very well on mild to moderate back pain. Those who suffer from ulcers and heartburn, however, should not use it." White willow bark can be purchased in capsule form from most health food stores.

The birch tree also has a medicinal effect for backaches. It contains methyl salicylate, which has analgesic properties, and was used in folk medicine to relieve the ache of rheumatism. Many pharmacists combine synthetic methyl salicylate with menthol in ointments designed to relieve the pain of osteoarthritis and lower back pain. It is best applied externally in the form of a hot poultice from the leaves, bark, and catkins. The methyl salicylate is absorbed through the skin. (See page 30 for more information on pain-relieving herbs.)

Chronic Pain

If your back pain is not acute, pinpointing the cause of it may not be as simple as it sounds. For some people, the pain might be the nagging reminder of an old football injury, but more likely the pain came on gradually, over a period of years. If that's the case, you have to find out what you've been doing for years that could cause the problem. And that's not always easy.

Many times back pain may be the result of a deformity present at birth, an infectious disease that is causing your bone structure to erode, or a food allergy. Sometimes the pain is due to simple arthritis or a calcium deficiency caused by an abnormality in the way that your body absorbs the mineral (common in postmenopausal women). All of these sound like serious problems that require the help of a doctor. While they can be, many times these problems can be cleared up at home with the proper treatment.

The Sitz Bath

If the pain you are suffering is relatively high up, causing a feeling of contraction, you may actually be suffering from kidney trouble. Had Tom Sawyer been suffering from this type of backache, instead of heartache, his aunt's attempt to cure the boy with a sitz bath may have been more successful. According to the *Dictionary of the Best Tips and Secrets for Better Health*, "back pains can often be caused by pressure exerted by a swollen kidney on the nerves that run parallel to the spine. A few horsetail sitz baths should solve the problem, since the kidneys usually respond very well to this plant."

To prepare a sitz bath, fill a bucket half full of fresh horsetail (or 100 grams of dried plant) and fill the rest of the bucket with water. Let the plant soak overnight. Then filter, reheat, and add to a bath filled with hot water (at least 104 degrees Fahrenheit).

Now, you're ready to get in. While sitting in the bath, keep your feet up out of the water so only your seat and lower back are immersed up to the kidneys. The parts of your body that are not immersed should be covered with towels to avoid catching cold. Plan to stay in the bath for 20 to 60 minutes.

If the pain is persistent, Annemarie Colbin recommends that you try cutting back on fermented foods that have a high salt content (beer, sauerkraut, miso, tempeh, etc.) or any other foodstuffs that stress the kidneys.

The Case of Vitamin Deficiency

In their book *Life Extension*, Durk Pearson and Sandy Shaw cite several cases where patients who suffered from chronic back pain were helped, if not cured, by vitamin supplementation. In one particular case, a businessman, Mr. V, was so debilitated by back pain that, at the age of 50, he could no longer participate in strenuous physical activities like water and snow skiing:

"The pain was ever-present. When he drove his car, he could not do so for more than 20 minutes at a time without developing intolerable back pain. So Mr. V purchased a station wagon and, when he traveled over 20 minutes or so, he would have to be chauffeured about lying on a foam rubber pad in the back of the station wagon. The six different doctors Mr. V consulted all told him that he would be disabled for the rest of his life.

"We told Mr. V about the beneficial effects of large doses of vitamins A, C, and E for life extension purposes, but said nothing to him about possible effects on his back. He immediately began taking 15,000 I.U. of vitamin A, several grams of vitamin C, and a couple of thousand units of E each day. About two months later, Mr. V telephoned to tell us that suddenly one day he had noticed that his back didn't hurt anymore! Then he began skiing again. He promptly reinjured his back in a skiing mishap, but more vitamins A, C, and E took care of his back again, and he was skiing again within a week. He was now able to frequently engage in snow and water skiing and travel without having to lie down. The pain would return within a week or two if he stopped taking the vitamins, but his back would be fine so long as he took them."

In another story with similar results, Durk Pearson related how his back problems were successfully treated with high doses of vitamins. Pearson was born with an abnormally curved spine and was told by a specialist that surgery probably wouldn't help much and might do more harm. The doctor explained that in order to correct the problem, Pearson would have to wear a large, troublesome back brace. Pearson decided that he would rather live with the pain than wear the brace.

Pearson said, "About two months after I started to take 50,000 I.U. of vitamin A and about 1200 I.U. of vitamin E and 3 grams of vitamin C per day, I suddenly realized that I had not had a backache for several days. The backache returned within a few days each time I discontinued the vitamins, and vanished within a day after restarting them. Although this was not a double-blind placebo-controlled test, I had *not* expected the vitamins to do anything for my bad back. I was taking the vitamins strictly for prophylaxis against free radical aging damage, which I thought would have only very long-term effects. Indeed, in 1968, I expected no perceptible short-term effects whatsoever, and was initially quite reluctant to ascribe the results to the vitamins. Moreover, I am not a strong placebo responder, and placebo effects rarely persist for long periods of time. Before using these large doses of antioxidant vitamins, I had had a chronic backache for over 20 years; with the vitamins, I have been normally free of backache...."

Backaches and Allergy

After suffering from a backache for several years, Mr. Dykstra paid a visit to Dr. Jonathan Wright. He explained to the doctor that he had seen seven chiropractors and four osteopaths, along with a number of other doctors and specialists, but none were able to help him.

His pain was a deep aching sensation within the muscles of his back. It started with leg aches and an occasional backache when he was six or seven. By the time he was 23 the aching in his back was steady. At the age of 37, the pain was centered in his back and "the only places that don't ache anymore are my hands, feet, and forearms. Even my calf muscles have started lately."

Dr. Wright asked if he suffered from any allergies or other illnesses when he was a child. Mr. Dykstra said that he did have an allergy to milk when he was two or three years old, but quickly outgrew it. He also mentioned that he had a problem with earaches.

With this information, Dr. Wright recommended that Mr. Dykstra eliminate all milk and dairy products from his diet. When Mr. Dykstra questioned the advice, Dr. Wright said, "Remember all those earaches you told me about? The vast majority of children with recurrent earaches are allergic to food.... Most allergic children with earaches quit having them after age four or so; the allergies simply switch symptoms or go 'underground.' I think yours switched to muscle aching. Remember, you've had that since you were six or seven."

When Mr. Dykstra eliminated the milk and dairy products from his diet, most of his muscle aching dissipated within a week. After having some allergy tests done, Mr. Dykstra stopped eating all the foods he was allergic to and his backache completely disappeared.

Dr. Wright said, "Dr. James C. Breneman, author of a basic textbook on food allergy, lists back pain as one of the common manifestations of food allergy.... Many individuals who 'outgrew' childhood allergies find that years later their allergies are still present, causing an entirely different set of symptoms....

"Except in cases of hypoglycemia (low blood sugar), serious underweight, or debilitating disease, a five-day fast (distilled water only) is often the quickest way to determine whether or not symptoms are caused by food sensitivity, including allergy. Younger children often can't

Climbing Out of Arthritis

"Perhaps 30 years ago, when I was climbing poles for a power company, I began experiencing pain in my elbow and shoulders. The misery would migrate from side to side, staying usually on a side several days before crossing to the other side. When I visited my doctor, he diagnosed it as gouty arthritis.

"At the time, I was eating several food supplements, including four tablets daily of alfalfa. I had heard of instances where alfalfa sometimes relieved the symptoms of some types of arthritis, so I increased my intake of alfalfa to six tablets in the morning and six at supper.

"After perhaps three months, my arthritis symptoms disappeared, returning only once when I went on a one-week fishing trip and didn't take my supplements along. About three to four days into the excursion, the pain returned and remained until I returned home and resumed consumption of the alfalfa. About four days later, the misery once again disappeared and I've had no recurrence since.

"Also, I once was bothered quite uncomfortably by fistulas. My doctor recommended hot water baths (which did help), but the fistulas kept returning. I was using a basic supplement at the time and decided to add vitamin E, vitamin C, zinc, calcium with magnesium, EPA, garlic, beta carotene, and, of course, alfalfa. The fistulas have never returned. I don't know which element effected the change, but I'm pretty happy about it. I suspect it was the vitamin E." — *D.W.D., Minnesota*

fast, either, but for most adults, such a fast will settle the question."

According to Dr. Wright, many chronic illnesses are the result of food allergies that are never diagnosed. If you have a malady that you can't get rid of, you may want to try Dr. Wright's recommendation of a five-day fast. The results just might surprise you.

Chapter 4

Those Annoying Aches and Pains

As we said in the introduction, pain is a very personal problem and usually requires a personal method of dealing with it. Besides the previously mentioned headaches and backaches, pain comes in many aggravating forms. There's arthritic pain, ocular pain, breast pain, rectal pain, menstrual pain, muscular and nervous pain, and osseous pain, to name just a few.

As we have seen in this report, both headaches and backaches can often times be relieved by the proper administration of plants and vitamins. Many of these same remedies are also effective for other types of pain.

For instance, Durk Pearson discussed the dramatic effects he has experienced using massive doses of vitamins A, C, and E for backache. These same types of effects were also seen in the treatment of arthritis, leg cramps, and varicose veins.

Dr. James Greenwood said in the *Dictionary of the Best Tips and Secrets for Better Health*, "The most spectacular effect of vitamin C is the way it prevents and soothes muscular pain due to excessive physical effort,

Arthritis Relief?

"Relief without side effects may be at hand for many arthritis sufferers. In a series of recent studies conducted at Indian government laboratories, the extract from Boswellia Serratta, a large branching tree that grows in dry hilly areas, was found to be both safe and effective....

"Researchers are showing that Boswellia is indeed potent for inflammatory diseases such as arthritis. It effectively shrinks inflamed tissue, the underlying cause of pain, by improving the blood supply to the affected area and enhancing the repair of local blood vessels damaged by proliferating inflammation....

"In one study conducted at the Government Medical College in Jammu, India, nearly 70 percent of arthritic patients tested experienced good to excellent re-sults against stiffness and pain. Over three-quarters of the patients in the study were either bedridden or incapacitated from doing normal work. Within two to four weeks after starting on the Boswellia extract, they reported a lessening of joint stiffness, pain, and improved grip strength....

"In the United States, physicians are giving Boswellia high marks for effectiveness. Dr. E.W. McDonagh, a Kansas City physician, has reported success among some 350 patients suffering from a variety of advanced muscular and skeletal conditions for whom other treatments had failed to help....

"There are no known major negative side effects from using Boswellia. One of the main U.S. distributors of Boswellia is Legere Pharmaceuticals (800-528-3144)." (*Women's Health Letter*, 1/94)

such as a long trek, an ocean voyage, a mountain climbing expedition, etc." But for the vitamin to work effectively, you have to take 1,500 milligrams a day before you are involved in the intense physical strain.

B complex vitamins are also recommended for soothing and treating pain. According to Dr. Richard M. Linchitz of the Pain Alleviation Centre of Long Island, vitamin B_3 "has been successful in treating arthritic pain and eliminating migraines." Also, vitamin B_6 "plays a role similar to that of vitamin B_3 in the production of anti-pain neurotransmitters. It also reinforces the immune system, which can become weakened from chronic pain."

Athletes and Fruit Juice

When active people begin having problems with pain in their joints, they often attribute the pain to overuse. Tennis players and baseball pitchers often complain of a malady called "tennis elbow." But you don't have to be a tennis player to suffer from this disorder. Many people suffer from a similar problem in their shoulders and hips.

The pain can be caused by an arthritic joint, tendonitis, bursitis, or deposits in the tissues. But Dr. George Meinig, in his book *"NEW"trition*, presents an alternative cause.

"Neuritis and bursitis are fancy diagnostic names we professionals give such problems, but the name only says one has inflammation present in these areas. It says nothing about the chemistry responsible for the pain....

"Orange juice is a common thirst quencher for tennis players. In my opinion, it is also the main reason for so many tennis elbows."

Most fruit drinks have a high content of acid, sugar, and potassium, which have a detrimental effect on the body's calcium/phosphorus balance (increase in calcium and a decrease in phosphorus). However, the increase in calcium in the blood stream is not taken from more food or supplementation. It is taken from the body's storage of calcium in the bones and teeth.

"On a hot day a tennis player has no trouble downing a pint to a quart or more of juice during a game. We must be aware that represents the juice of eight to 20 oranges. Heavy perspiration quickly uses the water in the juice, leaving the body to solve the chemistry problem created by the remaining high amounts of citric acid, sugar, and potassium, not to mention other ingredients in the fruit. The high concentration of these substances imbalances the normal mineral content. One of the principle problems is potassium has a thing about calcium. When too high it pulls out calcium from one's bones and teeth."

To solve the problem, simply stick to drinking water with a pinch of salt added. Most people don't get enough water, anyway, and the problem is compounded when they perspire heavily. Most people think that they get enough water from coffee, tea, juices, and soft drinks, but these are actually foods or chemicals that must enter the body's digestive mixture and usually leave the body dehydrated. Dr. William Campbell Douglass, editor of *Second Opinion*, warns that "heavy ingestion of high-sugar fruit juice is an invitation to adult-onset diabetes."

Treating Pain with Herbs

There's an old folk remedy from Louisiana that says you can transfer the pain of rheumatism to a tree in the middle of the forest. All you have to do, according to *American Folk Medicine*, is "follow a path in the woods where no one is likely to pass; when you reach the foot of a tree, any tree at all, dig up the root with your left hand and, holding the tree root between your teeth, say, 'Rheumatism, I leave you here and I will take you back when I pass this way again.' Then bury the root with your left hand. If you take care to avoid this spot in the future, a complete cure is guaranteed."

While we're not about to recommend this sort of superstitious mumbo-jumbo to you, the fact is there is much to be said for using trees, roots, and other plants to treat the pain and inflammation of rheumatism.

When it comes to herbal remedies, most medical doctors just smile with warm amusement and insist that if the treatment actually does work, it must be due to the placebo effect. But what these doctors won't admit is that many herbal remedies have been passed down from generation to generation for the simple reason that they *do* work.

Many times a headache, backache, and other types of pain can be treated very successfully with specific herbs. If you're an herb lover, and even if you're not, the following herbs might just be the thing your throbbing head is looking for. But be warned, not all of them will work for everybody and many will provide only temporary relief. Of course, if you're in pain, temporary relief is better than none at all. According to many experts, including *Rodale's Illustrated Encyclopedia of Herbs*, headache sufferers should try:

Alfalfa

A very popular herbal remedy for rheumatism that has been ignored by modern science is alfalfa. Most Westerners think of the common alfalfa plant as cattle fodder and, as a result, miss out on its beneficial health properties.

The herb can be taken in several different forms. The most convenient way is as a tablet or capsule, commonly available at most health food stores. Make sure to buy the large economy size; Dr. Earl Mindell says you'll need to take between nine and 18 tablets each day.

A "Shortened" Remedy for Bruises

"Anybody with kids knows that bruises are a fact of life. Well, I have twins, so I would have double the trouble if it weren't for my 'boo-boo cream.' Any time one of the girls bumps her head on the corner of the table, or whacks her shin on a chair, or whatever (seems like they always bump their forehead the day before their pictures are to be taken), I immediately apply some Crisco shortening. I don't know what it is, but it keeps bruises from forming after a hard knock. I've even had to use it on my husband a few times, with the same results. I've also found that butter flavored Crisco works just as well. But make sure you put in on immediately after the accident. If you wait too long, the magic disappears." — *J.T., Georgia*

You can also get your alfalfa by simply putting the sprouts in your favorite salad. But the most effective method is to make a tea. The following testimony from *Natural Home Remedies* explains how:

"I had arthritis for 11 years. The crippling kind, rheumatoid arthritis, spent a lot of money on it, including $500 at one doctor's office, and guess what completely cured me? Alfalfa tea, four or five glasses a day, every day. Now this is made with the seed, not the leaves. We have talked to so many people who have said, 'Oh I tried that and it didn't help' — and come to find out, they had tried the leaf tea. We all know the seeds have so much more in them than the leaves. Following is a recipe.

"Alfalfa Tea: Cook (not boil, so water is just moving), in an enamel or glass pan (not metal) with the lid on for one-half hour. Use one ounce alfalfa seed (untreated) with 1 1/4 pints water. After cooking, strain, squeezing or pressing seeds dry. Add honey to taste. Cool and put in refrigerator as soon as possible. Make up fresh daily. To use — mix strong base with one-half water (or to taste) for hot or cold tea. Use six or seven cups or four or five glasses a day. Try for at least two weeks." — A.G., Illinois.

There is one word of caution about alfalfa, though. It has been known to aggravate lupus and other auto-immune disorders. So if you have any problems with your immune system, avoid using this herb. I also wouldn't take the advice of my uncle who, upon hearing that my aunt was buying alphalfa tablets, asked, "Why don't you just run a rabbit through the alphalfa field? You'll get the same thing and it won't cost a dime."

Angelica

The medicinal use of angelica is largely focused on the treatment of digestive and bronchial problems. But when used in a decoction, the plant has been used successfully to treat nervous headaches and toothaches. Also, a teaspoon of the root or seeds boiled or steeped in a cup of water has been recommended by Michael Moore, author of *Medicinal Plants of the Mountain West*.

Arnica

The Germans use arnica in more than 100 drug preparations because of its ability to relieve pain. It is best used in an ointment to relieve the pain and inflammation of sprains and bruises. *Rodale's* said, "To make a liniment, heat 1 ounce of flowers in 1 ounce of lard or oil for several hours. Strain and let the ointment cool before applying it to bruises or sore muscles." The herb should not be used internally for self-treatment. It can be quite poisonous.

Basil

Like angelica, basil is recommended for digestive complaints and, if your headaches stem from constipation, this may explain the herb's effectiveness. However, basil also has a slight sedative action, which is why it is usually recommended for headaches. Pliny, the Roman author and philosopher, was one of the earliest to recommend basil tea as a remedy for headaches.

Betony

According to *Rodale's*, "A study done by scientists in the Soviet Union found that betony contains a mixture of glycosides, which showed some effect in lowering blood pressure. This might explain why infusions of betony have been recommended for headaches and mild anxiety attacks."

Birch

The leaves of the elegant birch tree contain methyl salicylate, which has counter-irritant and analgesic properties that help reduce the pain of rheumatism. The skin absorbs methyl salicylate very effectively, making birch a popular treatment today. Modern medicine uses synthetic methyl salicylate in many commercial creams and liniments to relieve the pain of various musculoskeletal conditions.

Lelord Kordel's *Natural Folk Remedies* describes a decoction of birch that can be used when the entire body aches. Kordel writes, "Place two pounds of fresh birch leaves (or one pound of dried) in a cotton bag or old pillowcase. Boil gently in two gallons of water for 40 minutes. Add both the bag and the birch water to a bathtub of comfortably hot water and soak for at least 20 minutes, adding more hot water as needed. (When birch leaves are not available, the same amount of pine needles make a relaxing, pain-easing substitute.)"

More Help for Arthritis

"This remedy for arthritis sounds too easy to be any good, but it really works! First, go to the store and buy one box of raisins, either golden or regular, and one bottle of gin (buy the cheapest you can find — I pay about $5 for a one-quart bottle). Then take the raisins and soak them in the gin for seven days. An old mayonnaise jar works great for this. Drain off the gin and take nine raisins daily.

"I've also got a quick-fix for hiccups. Simply massage your earlobe between your thumb and index finger. The hiccups will stop almost immediately. This sounds kinky, but it works." — *C.W.S., Colorado*

Blue Cohosh

The American Indians used blue cohosh, a deciduous, perennial plant, to reduce the pain and swelling of rheumatism. Ninety years ago, Dr. Josephus Goodenough explained in his *Home Cures and Herbal Remedies* how he used "a strong decoction of this plant, combined with slippery elm bark, to form a good poultice for every kind of inflammation."

Dr. Goodenough also combined "two ounces of the Cohosh root to one ounce of Blood Root infused in proof spirits and taken in wineglassful doses three times a day." A note of caution, however: if you have high blood pressure, avoid using blue cohosh, because it constricts the blood vessels of the heart.

Dr. Earl Mindell warns in his *Herb Bible* that large doses of cohosh can cause symptoms of poisoning and that it should not be used during pregnancy until labor begins (and then only under the supervision of a doctor). The herb is often used to induce labor.

Mindell says that one capsule should be taken up to three times per day. Or you can "mix 10 to 30 drops of extract in liquid daily."

Cabbage

Cabbage-leaf poultices can be applied to the back of the neck in order to combat headaches and other types of pain successfully.

Catnip

Called "Mother Nature's version of Alka-Seltzer," an infusion of catnip with chamomile and peppermint, sweetened with honey, is excellent for relieving symptoms of colds, headaches, and indigestion. In preparing the herb, make sure you don't boil it and don't drink more than a cup for each dose. Excessive doses can produce nausea.

Chamomile

Chamomile, or camomile, is famous for being one of the best natural analgesics. The *Dictionary of the Best Tips and Secrets for Better Health* says, "It has been used over the ages to combat pain from migraines, neuralgia, stomach or intestinal cramps, toothaches, muscle aches, rheumatism, bruises, difficult menstruation, liver disorders, colds, coughs, skin irritations, etc." The herb can be prepared for internal consumption by making an infusion with five to 10 flowers per cup. Drink three to four cups per day. You can also crush the flowers with a mortar and pestle and mix with equal amounts of honey to make a paste. You should take .35 to .7 oz. of the mixture three times each day. Applying ground chamomile leaves directly to inflamed skin areas helps reduce the swelling and tenderness.

Coffee

Caffeine is the principal active ingredient in coffee, aspirin, and many modern analgesics. That explains why coffee is often used to battle migraine headaches.

Comfrey

Also can be used for inflammation, especially around cuts, sores, insect bites and stings, burns, etc. According to *1,001 Home Health Remedies*, "Grinding the leaves in a blender makes an ointment that you can rub directly on the skin to help reduce pain and swelling."

Devil's Claw

The root of the devil's claw is said to be one of the most extraordinary plants in existence for fighting rheumatism and arthritis. The *Dictionary of the Best Tips and Secrets for Better Health* lists three ways you can effectively use devil's claw root. The first, and probably the most convenient, is to buy devil's claw root tablets at your local health food store. Take up to three grams per day.

The second consists of preheating your teapot and then adding "a teaspoon of dried root and half a quart of boiling water. Let the mixture cool down as slowly as possible (by placing the teapot next to a heat source). Let it soak overnight. Then filter and drink three cups per day.

And finally, "you can make your own devil's claw root ointment" by filling a bowl with devil's claw root (don't press it together) and covering it with sweet almond oil. Let it stand for two weeks and then filter. To the oil, add 1.4 fl. oz. of hot wax per half quart of oil. "Mix well and pour into containers with large openings. Apply to affected areas. You will find the ointment extremely effective."

Echinacea

Taking one tablespoon of a decoction of echinacea three to six times a day is an effective treatment for headaches and many other ailments. With a compress, it can also be used on wounds and painful swellings.

Fennel

Has a reputation for curing headaches caused by bad digestion when eaten raw or cooked.

Feverfew

In 1980, scientists confirmed in the British medical journal *Lancet* that feverfew, which has long been used against migraines, shares many properties with aspirin. Varro Tyler, Ph.D., dean of the school of Pharmacy, Nursing, and Health Sciences at Purdue University, says, "If you take feverfew by eating the leaves, it should be in very small doses — from 50 to 60 milligrams, which is three or four of the little feverfew leaves each day." Many people mix the leaves into food to hide the bitter taste and some botanical wholesalers sell the herb in capsule form. It has been used very effectively on migraines.

Garlic

Excellent for relieving the pain of insect bites and stings. Just rub the clove directly on the sting or bite.

Ginger

"You may be able to reach into your kitchen spice cabinet for relief from the pain and inflammation of rheumatoid arthritis," says the *Book of Proven Home Remedies and Natural Healing Secrets*. "People with arthritis reported 'significant relief' from pain after taking less than a tablespoonful of ginger every day for three months, reports Dr. Krishna C. Srivastava of the Institute of Odense in Denmark. Long known as a folk remedy for various ailments, ginger now is being studied in medical trials to determine its usefulness as an arthritis medicine.

"The arthritis patients took ginger in two ways: either about five grams a day of fresh gingerroot, or from a half-gram to 1.5 grams daily of ginger powder.

"All reported that 'they were able to move around better and had less swelling and morning stiffness after taking the spice,' says the *Medical Tribune* (30,18:16). No side effects were reported."

Goldenrod

The European goldenrod is prepared in Chinese medicine as a headache remedy. However, if you're allergic to pollen, it would be best to stay away from goldenrod.

Horseradish

You probably think that horseradish is a sauce or spice, but herb specialists have long been using it in the treatment of digestion. *The Book of 1,001 Home Health Remedies* says, "This member of the mustard family can also be used as a pain relieving remedy for neck and back pain. Or you can use a gargle mixture of grated horseradish, honey, and water as a way to ease hoarseness." Horseradish poultices can be applied to the back of the neck in order to combat headaches successfully.

Lavender

Lavender has only modest abilities as a medicinal herb, but it has been used to relieve headaches and toothaches. Works best by massaging your temples with a couple of drops of the essence.

Lettuce

Common garden lettuce eaten in a salad is an effective herb to use for pain. It has a sedative effect that is very similar to opium, but doesn't have the side effects.

Linden

Headaches that are a result of colds or flu can usually be alleviated by drinking linden flower infusions. Use approximately 1/6 oz. of linden per cup of boiling water and drink three to four cups per day. You can also slit the linden tree in the spring and use its sap. Three tablespoons of sap per day should do the trick.

Lovage

Some Europeans use this herb as a folk cure for headaches.

Onion

The bulb of the onion has several medicinal uses, but when eaten raw is especially good for the blood. You can also prepare a compress by mixing two pureed onions with olive oil and salt and applying it to the painful area. Also works well for bruises and sprains. Onion poultices can be applied to the back of the neck in order to combat headaches successfully.

Oregano

Most modern herbalists recommend infusions of oregano leaves to treat headaches. The leaves can also be used externally in a warm poultice to soothe painful swellings.

Peppermint

Applying freshly gathered and crushed peppermint leaves to the forehead is an effective headache remedy. The leaves may also be used to soothe tired, sore muscles, or arthritic joints. To relieve the pressure of sinus headaches, place 5-10 drops of peppermint oil into two quarts of hot water and gently inhale the vapors. And rubbing the oil on the skin gives a soothing sensation for aching muscles and joints. Peppermint tea is also good for the sinuses and menstrual cramps.

Poplar

The poplar genus shares many of the same properties as common aspirin. Therefore, any ailment that you would normally use aspirin to treat will probably respond in much the same way with the internal use of poplar medications.

Rosemary

For headache pain, use a couple of drops of rosemary essence to massage the temples. This may also work for rheumatism and bruises.

Sage

This member of the mint family is extraordinary in its ability to relieve sore throats, mouth and gum problems, cuts and sores, bruises, and other skin problems.

Thyme

Most herbalists use a warm infusion of thyme to treat headaches. Also, a poultice made by mashing the leaves into a paste is effective on inflammation and sores.

Willow

According to the *Dictionary of the Best Tips and Secrets for Better Health*, the "white willow is called the 'pain tree' because it was used so often by healers to treat fever before quinine was invented. It is rich in salicin, a glucoside contained in its bark." When medical science finally caught up to this folk remedy, the world was introduced to aspirin. As is so often the case, medical science was unable to improve upon God's creation and produced a pill that causes bleeding in the digestive tract.

But you can still use willow bark very effectively to treat rheumatism and other aches and pains (such as headaches). Herbalist Michael Weiner, in his book *Weiner's Herbal*, recommends that you make a decoction of one teaspoon white willow bark boiled slowly for 30 minutes in 1 1/2 pints of water in a covered container. After slowly cooling, drink the decoction a tablespoonful at a time as needed.

You can also make a tea out of the bark to drink as you need it. Or simply chew on a piece of willow bark to release its natural pain-killers.

As you can see there are many effective ways to treat your pain with herbs. Some people have reported complete cures with continued use of these remedies, while others receive temporary relief.

Conclusion

For most people, pain doesn't have to be a way of life. Our body was created with the ability to heal itself, but many times our bad habits inhibit the body from doing its job. Some of our habits only cause minor problems that we can live with, while others can be crippling and even life-threatening.

Annemarie Colbin sums it up quite well: "If we panic at a headache or fever and suppress them with aspirin, if we worry about a minor infection and cart out the antibiotic artillery, we often get ourselves into a worse state simply out of fear. But if we welcome minor disturbances as early warning signals pointing out our mistakes and learn to interpret them, we will have plenty of time to make corrections and thereby avoid the escalation and aggravation of our health problems.

"Because the body tends to heal itself if allowed to do so, most of the time all we have to do is get out of the way and let it carry on. Thus, through rest, fasting, appropriate food selection, and a few gentle nudges from natural remedies, we can easily regain our equilibrium and thereby stand a good chance of functioning joyfully and actively for many years."

When Tom Sawyer was hurting, his aunt finally gave him some "Painkiller." The alcohol content instantly bettered the boy's disposition, but it wasn't until Tom "felt that it was time to wake up" that he decided to think "over various plans for relief."

It wasn't the Painkiller that cured Tom, it was his change in attitude. For physical pain, that's the first step.

Chapter 5

Questions and Answers

Gout

Q. I've suffered from gout for some time now and was wondering if you had any suggestions on how to deal with this terrible pain?

A. If your big toe is in severe pain, you might understand these words written by the English writer and Anglican priest Sydney Smith: "Oh! When I have the gout I feel as if I was walking on my eyeballs." These words were written back in the early 1800s when gout was thought to be a Divine Right of Kings.

But through the years, gout has become a problem that afflicts more than just the aristocrats. Today, over 1.6 million Americans, primarily men, suffer with this unduly painful malady.

If you have gout, your body is either producing too much uric acid or is not excreting enough of it. When this happens, sharp microscopic crystals of sodium urate begin to develop around and prick the joint tissue. For some reason, the joint of the big toe seems to be a favorite target of the crystals.

Gout was long considered a disease of the wealthy because it is usually caused by an excessively rich diet, which only the wealthy could afford. As the diet of more people began to include rich foods, gout slowly became a bigger problem. Foods that are rich in purines (substances found in high-protein foods), such as anchovies, asparagus, liver, sardines, and mussels, are delicacies in many countries, but have become popular with the average citizen in the U.S.

Modern medicine has shown that the body's inability to metabolize purines is the main reason for the excess uric acid. While they probably had no idea what a purine was as early as the 18th century, many people knew that rich meals and gout were somehow related. They had a pretty good idea that alcohol was also part of the problem.

To relieve the pain, these early medical pioneers knew that restricting the foods they ate and avoiding alcohol was the best form of treatment. But they also discovered something else. Dr. Goodenough explains his treatment for chronic gout in his book *Home Cures and Herbal Remedies*, "Take hot vinegar and put into it all the table salt which it will dissolve, and bathe the parts affected with a soft piece of flannel. Rub in with the hand, and dry the part by the fire. Repeat this operation four times in 24 hours, 15 minutes each time, for four days; then twice a day for the same period; then once, and follow this rule whenever the symptoms show themselves at any future time."

Another age-old remedy for gout was found deep in the Amazon jungles of Brazil where natives had been using a natural tonic for as long as three centuries. In

Brazil, the tonic is known as *para todo*, but sells in the U.S. as a dietary supplement called "Suma."

According to the book *Amazing Medicines the Drug Companies Don't Want You to Discover!*, University of Sao Paolo professor of pharmacology Dr. Milton Brazzach "found [Suma] was not a cure, but brought significant relief for ... gout sufferers, with no undesirable side effects. And doses as low as one gram a day produced basic feelings of well-being." Suma can be purchased at most health food and vitamin stores.

Gout is a disease that, while painful, can be easily controlled and even cured in many cases. Isn't it good to know that you can stop walking on your eyeballs?

Carpal Tunnel Syndrome

Q. I've been a secretary for eight years and have often suffered pain in my wrists. My doctor tells me that it's a condition called carpal tunnel syndrome and may require surgery to relieve the pain. Is there something I can do at home to avoid the surgery?

A. Carpal tunnel syndrome is a neurological disease that is caused by repetitive motions in certain types of work in offices and factories. It is characterized by numbness, pain, and tingling in the involved hand or fingers. Patients who suffer with this syndrome may also have a weak grip and muscle spasms during the night. Brief paralysis can also occur.

According to the Oregon State University newsletter ("OSU This Week," 3/17/94), OSU researchers have shown that vitamin B_6 will often relieve the symptoms of CTS. Doctors in the field of nutritional therapy have been prescribing B_6 for this condition for 20 years. A dose of 50 to 100 mg per day should work, if it's going to work. Some doctors recommend taking dosages as high as 300 mg per day for severe or stubborn cases. It's not successful in every case, but it certainly should be tried before surgery.

Huntington's Disease

Q. I am writing to ask for information regarding 'Huntington's Disease' and if there is any treatment with vitamins and supplements that can help a patient.

A. Huntington's disease is thought to be a hereditary disease of the central nervous system that is characterized by progressive dementia and rapid, jerky motions. Modern medicine insists that there is no cure for this disease, but wholistic physicians have seen the symptoms completely abate in many cases.

Currently, there are two supplements that have enjoyed a great deal of success in the treatment of Huntington's disease. The first is called choline. Researchers are finding that choline can be extremely helpful in some diseases that result in abnormal muscular movements. Choline is available from most health food stores.

The other supplement that has been used to treat Huntington's disease successfully is DMAE. This nutrient is found most abundantly in the "brain" foods, such as anchovies and sardines. According to the book *Amazing Medicines the Drug Companies Don't Want You to Discover*, "DMAE has the remarkable ability to cross the blood-brain barrier. Subsequent experiments have shown that the nutrient is responsible for extending the life spans of animals by approximately 30 to 40 percent."

DMAE is available in a product called Gero Vita GH3 from Gero Vita Laboratories, 1350 E. Flamingo Road, Dept. Z100, Las Vegas, NV 89119, 800-825-8482. One doctor said, "An average of 1,000 mg daily in adults seems to be necessary for achieving clear cut therapeutic effects. The best clinical effects have been achieved after three months of treatment."

Neuralgia

Q. I am a rather healthy person (over the age of 65), but I now have neuralgia. I am able to control the pain myself without medicine. The neuralgia clears up for weeks at a time, then it flares up again. I don't know what triggers the flare-ups. I can stand the pain, but any help you might offer would be greatly appreciated.

A. Neuralgia is caused by the irritation of a nerve and is usually accompanied by spasms of pain along the course of the nerve. The irritation can come from a variety of sources — lack of a proper diet, dental decay, eye strain, exposure to dampness and cold with a resulting infection, or any other type of infection. And the pain can be accompanied by muscle weakness, paralysis, or numbness of the skin.

There are several types of neuralgias, each affecting a different part of the body, with the most common being Bell's palsy and trigeminal neuralgia. A case of Bell's palsy recently hit a young lady in our office while she was pregnant. The left side of her face was completely para- lyzed, causing her cheek to droop and her eye to dry out and become irritated. It also slurred her speech and made eating and drinking very difficult. It was a miserable time for her, but she was a trooper.

Fortunately, this malady has an 80 percent recovery rate and is not accompanied by a great deal of pain. Within a few weeks, our colleague had made a complete recovery, just in time for the holidays, and has suffered no other symptoms.

But other cases of neuralgia are not so fortunate. We recently received the following letter from a subscriber:

"I have read several booklets and subscribed to health letters hoping to find a cure for my trigeminal neuralgia. It is confined to an area above the extreme left side of my upper lip. The condition has persisted for about 10 years with it worsening recently.

"I had gone to a neurologist who tried Tegretol and Dilantin on me. Being allergic to both medications, I couldn't pursue that method. He referred me to a neurosurgeon who wanted to inject alcohol into the focal point. I would have to endure a numb left side of my face permanently. I wouldn't go for that.

"Is there any cure for my condition?" — *C.T., Michigan*

Most doctors would answer this gentleman's question with a resounding "No." But through the years, other doctors and nutritionists have been courageous enough to challenge the wisdom of the establishment.

Jethro Kloss, in his book *Back to Eden*, recommends the use of "hot and cold compresses to the painful area when the flare-ups occur. The cold portion of the treatment must be kept very short. A hot fomentation wrung out of a tea made of mullein and lobelia and applied to the affected parts, will do much to relieve the pain. Herbal liniment, applied freely and rubbed in thoroughly, will relieve the pain in a short time....

"To make herbal liniment, combine two ounces powdered myrrh, one ounce powdered golden seal, one-half ounce cayenne pepper, and one quart rubbing alcohol (70 percent). Mix together and let stand seven days; shake well every day, decant off, and bottle in corked bottles. If you do not have golden seal, make the liniment without it (be careful not to get it into the eye)."

And he adds, "Placing the opposite hand and arm in very hot water for 20 minutes will frequently give relief.... Daily massage to the area is very helpful. Rest in bed and a nourishing diet, including adequate vitamin E, are essential."

Dr. Josephus Goodenough explained in his book *Home Cures and Herbal Remedies* that neuralgic "conditions are evidence that there remains in the system irritating waste material that should be eliminated. As evidence that these statements are true, these cases almost universally give a history of constipation. The urine is highly colored ... due to uric acid, which has been rasping through the system and which the kidneys are doing their best to eliminate. Sick headache is also an evidence of indigestion followed by the production of poison that produces local irritation in the stomach. The undigested food also aids or increases the irritation."

Goodenough continued, "Let us view the situation from another standpoint. The circulation of the brain is conducted through the carotid arteries. These are situated one on either side of the neck, and lie parallel to the jugular vein. The one on the left side is more direct, hence it is shorter. The result is a more forcible circulation, resulting in greater pressure, and it follows that any irritating substances or material would produce a sharper or more acute effect. This explains [why] neuralgia of the face usually occurs on the left side."

To help speed the elimination of toxins, says Goodenough, "take English Valerian, steep to make a tea and drink freely of it...." Fasting is also beneficial for freeing the body of these poisons. Externally, Goodenough recommends "counter-irritants, such as mustard plasters, etc., placed over the region of pain."

In 1937, Drs. Edward H. Kotin and David Stein reported in the *New York Physician* that garlic can be used very effectively as another counter-irritant. For the purpose of treating neuralgia they found it advantageous to use garlic in the compress form.

In 1960, Dr. R. Swinburne Clymer gave the following recipe in *The Medicines of Nature*: A compound tincture of two ounces of myrrh and a half-ounce of capsicum is a powerful external application for neuralgia. To make it even more potent, add four ounces of echinacea.

Two other herbs that have been successful at easing the pain of neuralgia are black cohosh and white willow bark. These herbs are generally accepted as treatments for rheumatism and, because neuralgia is essentially a form of rheumatism, they work well for the treatment of neuralgia. You can buy these herbs in capsule form at your local health food store. If you use black cohosh, take one capsule up to three times daily. Or if you prefer white willow bark, take two capsules every two to three hours as needed.

When the pain from neuralgia reaches a sudden crisis, Dr. H.C.A. Vogel recommends the homeopathic medicine *Belladonna 4x*. He explains in his book, *The Nature Doctor*, "It is important to keep belladonna in your medicine chest; if used at once when needed, many a serious problem can be avoided.... Auntie may be troubled by sudden neuralgic pains ... she will find relief from five drops of belladonna taken in a small glass of water. This first aid rarely fails."

Another quick-fix for that sudden onslaught of neuralgic pain is found in Gipsy Petulengro's book, *Romany Remedies and Recipes*. This authentic gypsy recipe calls for one ounce of the herb ladies' slipper root boiled in one pint of water for 10 minutes. Strain and bottle the liquid. When the attack hits take a wineglassful and then take the same dose as a sleep-inducer before retiring to bed.

It should be noted that most quick-fixes for neuralgia are just temporary, so attention to diet, elimination, fresh air, and proper exercise are all of the greatest importance. The following testimonial from *Natural Home Remedies* gives evidence:

"For 12 years I've had trigeminal neuralgia, and there seems to be no cure unless an operation is done. At first, the attack would last a few weeks, then go away. But through the years they've gotten stronger and now if I'm free of pain for a month or six weeks, it's unusual. I'm now on Dilantin; it doesn't cure, but does make the pain bearable.

"Do you know what gives me complete relief? Walking! I can't eat breakfast in the morning, as the pain is very acute when I first wake up. So I get outside and walk for an hour. Within the first 10 minutes, the pain is gone. And nothing that I do — bite, chew, talk, etc. — will bring that pain back. There are days when I 'walk my legs off.'" — *E.B.I., New York*

Many cases of neuralgia are caused by food allergies or sensitivities, so careful diet precautions must be taken. Jean Carper reported in her book *Food: Your Miracle Medicine* that a woman eliminated the "pain of neuralgia by giving up caffeine...."

According to Carper, the woman "regularly drank three to four cups of instant coffee a day, and drank more when the pain was particularly bad. Wondering if caffeine might be partly at fault, she switched to decaf. Remarkably, after two or three weeks the severe pain lessened.... For a whole year she remained free of episodes of pain by avoiding caffeine.... Later she noticed that a mere one cup of caffeinated coffee was enough to trigger a week-long episode of 'moderately intense' pain."

Another diet recommendation includes the elimination of high arginine foods, such as chocolate and nuts, from the diet. Researchers say that the herpes virus might be associated with some cases of neuralgia and this amino acid stimulates the virus.

Hopefully, one of these suggestions will cure your neuralgia, but if not, maybe one of them will help ease the pain of this terrible problem. If one of them works for you, please let me know.

Heel Spurs

Q. A couple of years ago I developed heel spurs from several years of walking golf courses and jogging. I've been to a local podiatrist, who periodically gives me cortisone shots in both heels. These shots provide comfort for a few months, then the pain becomes increasingly greater until additional cortisone is required. I need help — do you have any suggestions?

A. The best "at-home" treatment for a bone spur is vitamin C. The following testimonial from *Natural Home Remedies* should convince you of that.

"Several years ago, I suffered pain in my right heel, every time I put the foot down. It was very painful. I consulted a general practitioner and was told I most likely had a heel spur. The doctor prescribed pills and ointment which did not bring any relief....

"I was desperate. Only a person who has suffered a heel spur himself can know what that means. However, at that time I had read that in some cases of arthritis vitamin C is of help. I started wondering if there was any similarity between a heel spur and arthritis. I bought 250-milligram tablets of vitamin C and started ingesting them at the rate of 4,000 to 5,000 milligrams per day. On the third day in the afternoon the heel was not painful to lean on anymore and only slightly painful for about two weeks when pressed hard with a finger."

Ankylosing Spondylitis

Q. Do you have information on ankylosing spondylitis? My brother-in-law, age 40, suffers terribly from this disease and his doctor has been unable to help him. I've talked to and written several doctors and no one seems to have anything that helps.

A. Ankylosing spondylitis is a rare rheumatologic condition that causes partial or complete rigidity and inflammation of the spine and sacroiliac joints. The disease tends to strike only males in the 20 to 40 year old age range and it is characterized by a posture that is usually bent forward.

Some doctors have treated ankylosing spondylitis successfully by implementing a whole-foods diet with an emphasis on variety and ruling out allergies to certain foods. Alan R. Gaby, M.D. has found that identifying and avoiding allergic foods is extremely important for treatment. Many times, the health of the digestive system may be related to the disease. "Researchers at King College Hospital in London have found a link between ankylosing spondylitis and bowel dysbiosis (incursion or overgrowth by undesirable bacteria, in this case klebsiella). They discovered that the majority of patients placed on a low-starch diet had the disease process halted.

"Leon Chaitow, N.D., D.O., of London, England, feels that an overgrowth of *Candida albicans* (a naturally occurring fungus in the body) is also involved in creating the damage to the gastrointestinal tract which allows the klebsiella bacteria to enter the bloodstream. He recommends further measures, including the use of friendly bacteria such as acidophilus and bulgaricus to reestablish a normal bowel flora, and an anti-candida approach, which includes a low-fat diet. He believes that the results of the low-fat diet in the King College Hospital study may have been due to controlling both the klebsiella bacteria and the candida...."

"Many anti-inflammatory and alternative herbs have been used to alleviate the symptoms of this condition. The following mixture has been used over long periods of time: a combination of the tinctures of meadowsweet, willow bark, black cohosh, prickly ash, celery seed, and nettle in equal parts, one-half teaspoonful of this mixture taken three times a day. In cases of rheumatoid arthritis, add wild yam and valerian to the mixture and take one teaspoonful of this mixture three times a day."

(*Alternative Health*, Future Medicine Publishing, Inc., 1993)

To help digestive problems, drink two cups of vegetable broth daily. Other dietary considerations include vitamin C supplementation (eight to 10 grams daily) and the complete avoidance of sugar and alcohol. Yeast thrives on sugar in order to grow, so a low-sugar diet will help defeat the growth of candida. Alcohol should be avoided because it is composed of fermented and refined sugar.

Peripheral Neuropathy

Q. Many of my female friends and myself, ages 60 to 70, are experiencing numbness, burning, tingling, and odd sensations in our ankles and feet. Doctors call it peripheral neuropathy and say nothing can be done! Please help!

A. Peripheral neuropathy is a general reference to a disturbance in the peripheral nervous system (nerves outside of the spine). It is usually accompanied by spasms of pain along the course of the nerve, especially in the feet and ankles and even up to the thigh. The disturbance is usually noninflammatory in nature and is often the result of nutritional deficiencies.

Your doctors say that nothing can be done, but chances are they haven't tried everything. Many people have found relief from their symptoms simply by taking nutritional supplements. These supplements include thiamine (100 mg two to three times daily) and folic acid (500 mcg two times daily), along with niacin, vitamins C, B_6, B_{12}, and E, calcium, magnesium, lecithin, and brewer's yeast.

Unfortunately, as we grow older, our ability to absorb the right amount of vitamins and minerals can become less than efficient. There have been numerous studies showing that the body's ability to secrete gastric acid decreases with age. If the nutritional supplements listed above fail to give you relief, you should have a nutritionally oriented doctor check to see if your stomach is producing enough acid. If not, you will need to take a hydrochloric acid (HCl) supplement (see page 224 for HCl supplementation protocol) to help resolve the problem. It's truly amazing how many health problems are caused by this one problem.

In the meantime, try placing the opposite foot in very hot water for 20 minutes. This is an old folk remedy that has been known to give some temporary relief. Also, a daily massage to the area can be very helpful. And don't forget to get enough rest in bed and a nourishing diet. These are essential.

Bone Fractures

Q. A friend of mine told me the other day that giving soft drinks to my daughter on a daily basis is bad for her bones. Is this true?

A. Listen to your friend. Dr. Earl Mindell reported in the May 1995 issue of *Let's Live* some very negative news for soft drink consumers. He said, "Surveys were sent to 76 girls and 51 boys asking them about their medical histories and the frequency with which they drink soft drinks — colas and non-colas. A distinct relationship was found between cola beverage consumption and bone fractures in females. If the females had a high calcium intake, there was some protection. However, no association was found between non-cola soft drinks and bone fractures. Cola drinks are high in phosphoric acid, which can cause calcium to leave bones faster — a major risk factor for osteoporosis in postmenopausal women."

Section 2

Respiratory Problems

Chapter 6

Can Water Help Asthma Sufferers?

One of the most exciting days of the school year when I was growing up was Field Day. It was the Olympics of our elementary school, and we competed in everything from the three-legged race to the shoe kick to the egg toss. But the highlight of the day was the relay race. The whole school watched as the fastest four sixth-graders raced against four fleet-footed teachers (the teachers were always anchored by the principal, so it was an awesome thing to beat their team — a feat that hadn't been accomplished in years).

My final year of elementary school was especially electrifying, because we knew the teachers were nervous. We had Scott, one the fastest kids Maple Grove Elementary had seen in some time, not to mention three other students who weren't exactly slow.

During the first three legs of the race, the teachers were ahead, but only by a nose. We knew we had them! It was a magical moment when the third leg handed off to the anchors; it pitted Scott against our principal, and they were neck and neck at the handoff. Dr. Nocton got a quick jump, but Scott quickly made up the distance, passed the competition, and won the race by a commanding distance. We were ecstatic! Our principal lifted Scott up to his shoulders and joined in the celebration.

Asthma Linked to Polyunsaturated Oils

"Is there a link between childhood asthma and the consumption of polyunsaturated oils like safflower and sunflower oils? The authors conclude the increase in childhood asthma is due at least partially to the increased consumption of polyunsaturated oils and margarine.

"These oils are rich in omega 6 fatty acids, but low in omega 3 fatty acids. As the omega 6 fatty acids are metabolized, they produce a pro-inflammatory substance that can cause smooth muscle spasms. Therefore, they conclude the increase in omega 6 and the low intake of omega 3 fatty acids have led to the greater chance of asthma inflammation and constriction of the bronchial tubes. The greater use of polyunsaturated oils in Australia has led to an increase in childhood asthma.

"Similar statistics have been observed in New Zealand, the United Kingdom, and the United States. The probable reason for the shift to polyunsaturated oils, especially margarines, was the health benefit campaigns so well promoted in all of these countries." (*Australian New Zealand Journal of Medicine*, 1994; 24: 727; *Let's Live*, July 1995)

I remember that day vividly, because it was a day of triumph. Not only for the students, but for Scott. He suffered from asthma. He helped win the race, but the very fact that he could run without having a major asthma attack was an even bigger victory.

Back then, asthma was not that common — or at least I didn't think so. I had never heard of the disease until I met Scott in the fourth grade. But today the situation is much different. I have several friends who are elementary school teachers, and every one of them tells me that asthma is a major problem for many of the children in their classes.

If you or someone you love has asthma, you've probably read the grim statistics: There are now more than 10 million Americans that suffer from asthma; a 50 percent increase since 1980. The Centers for Disease Control estimates that one in every 20 persons is affected with the disease. It is the number one cause of absenteeism for elementary age children, and reported deaths due to asthma jumped 68 percent during the 1980s. A similar trend has been noted in several other industrialized countries, including Canada, England, Sweden, Denmark, and Australia.

Is There Any Relief?

As you can see by Scott's relatively normal life, asthma has been temporarily controlled in many instances by modern medicine. However, studies are now showing that many of the medications used by asthmatics can be quite dangerous. Scott used a bronchodilator that allowed him to participate in the normal activities of children. But now, researchers have found that heavy reliance on certain bronchodilator sprays increases the risk of dying from asthma by 40 times. And other asthma medicines are causing similar problems; some not as drastic, some worse.

Now that we're finding modern medicine isn't always the panacea we are told, is there any safe relief for the asthmatic?

The answer for many people is yes. We said last year that "new research from the University of Arizona is indicating that all cases of asthma are caused by allergies." So whether you're five, 35, or 75, there is more than likely a remedy, if not a cure, for your problem.

Back to Basics

You'll notice that I mention several times in this book the importance of drinking plenty of water. You already know that water is vitally important to your well-being. But do you know what happens when your body doesn't get enough water? One doctor's research indicates that numerous diseases are the direct result of a "settled-in dehydration." That includes many cases of asthma.

Water is the primary agent in the processes that take place in your body. You can name just about any function in the human body and water is involved somehow. Whether it be digestion or breathing, water is there. At birth, a baby is 85 percent water. The kidneys have a 40 mile network of filtration tubes that process 100 gallons of water a day. During the process, urine is strained out with its waste and the purified liquid is returned to the blood stream to benefit the body.

Since the introduction of soft drinks, mass-produced juices and teas, and Kool-Aid, Americans have gradually reduced the amount of pure water they consume each day. The results are devastating.

"Asthma and allergies are indicators that the body has resorted to an increase in production of the neurotransmitter histamine that is the sensor regulator of water metabolism and its distribution in the body," says Dr. F. Batmanghelidj, author of *Your Body's Many Cries for Water*.

He continued: "It is recognized that asthmatics have an increase in histamine content of their lung tissue and that it is the histamine that regulates the bronchial muscle contraction. Since one of the sites for water loss through evaporation is in the lungs, the bronchial constriction produced by histamine means less water evaporation during the act of breathing — *a simple natural maneuver to preserve the body water.*" (Emphasis added.)

"If you suffer from asthma or allergies, increase your daily water intake (to eight to 12 glasses a day, depending on your body weight). *Do not overdrink thinking you can undo the damage of many months or years of dehydration by excessive intake of water in a few days. You need to drink a normal amount every day until full hydration of the body is achieved over a longer period of time.*" (Emphasis in the original.)

Dr. Batmanghelidj also recommends decreasing the amount of orange juice asthmatics drink to one glass a day. "The potassium content of orange juice is high. High loads of potassium in the body can promote more than usual histamine production.... Although orange juice contains water, it cannot be assumed it replaces the needs of the body for pure and simple water."

Many asthmatics who have gone on diets that require drinking a lot of water (like the Jenny Craig diet) have found that their asthma symptoms decreased sharply. They may attribute their discovery to the diet, but don't be fooled, it was the water.

Soft Water or Hard?

If you take the word of advertisements, you might think that water softeners are the greatest thing to come along in years. But if you look at the scientific research you'll see just the opposite is true. Carol Zepp recently wrote in *Total Health*: "De-mineralized water (distilled and reverse osmosis processed) has 85-99 percent of everything removed including minerals. This type of water is then termed 'aggressive,' meaning it will seek out minerals to electro-magnetically balance itself! Anyone drinking this type of water must know that the water will pull minerals from the body."

Why is this important information for asthmatics? Researchers have performed biopsies on the lungs of asthmatics and found *significant vitamin and mineral deficiencies*. In fact, a new study reported in the *Lancet* (1994; 344:357-62) found that a 100-mg-a-day higher intake of magnesium was associated with an 18 percent reduction in the risk of hyperactivity and a 15 percent decrease in self-reported wheezing.

Therefore, asthmatics should not only drink eight to 12 glasses of water every day, but they should drink water with a high degree of calcium and magnesium. That means *hard* water. It's important to get these minerals from water because food may contain some chelating agents that prevent immediate absorption of certain elements. The food may contain high amounts of the element, but the body's actual percentage of absorption may be relatively small.

If you live in an area where the water is softened or polluted, start taking mineral supplements (you may want to take them even if you drink hard water). A daily regimen of 1,000 mg of vitamin C, 10,000 IU of beta carotene, 400 IU of vitamin E, and up to 500 mg of magnesium should help considerably. (A word of caution: If you have kidney trouble, check with a nutritionally oriented doctor before taking magnesium at these levels.) Health food stores have a capsule that combines magnesium, orotate, and glycinate and is very effective for asthmatics (take 500 mg per day).

If drinking more water doesn't ease your asthma symptoms, keep drinking the eight to 12 glasses a day. You'll be amazed at how much better you will feel.

Chapter 7

Treating Emphysema with Vitamins and Herbs

Emphysema is a health problem that very few home remedy books are willing to tackle. And rightly so. The disease is so complicated that most of the things you can do at home are more for coping with emphysema than for curing it. However, if you learn to properly cope with the disease, there's no reason you can't live a long, healthy life — especially if you begin treating it in its early stages.

If you do have emphysema, your doctor undoubtedly has told you to stop smoking. Smoking, after all, is the number one cause of emphysema. Once it is stopped, any therapy will be much more effective.

Smoking, along with automobile exhaust, supplies the lungs with large quantities of nitrous oxide, a poisonous gas that harms the lungs. The smoke from cigarettes destroys the oxygen-carrying capacity of hemoglobin (the substance that carries oxygen in the blood) and is also a major source of free radicals which, among other things, make the tissues in your lungs stiff and brittle. If caught in the early stages, a continued loss of flexibility in the

Fish Diet Protects Against Emphysema, Bronchitis

"Eyal Shahar, a University of Minnesota epidemiologist, and his colleagues quizzed 9,000 smokers and former smokers — those most at risk for lung disease — about their eating habits and overall health. About 900 said they had bronchitis or emphysema. After reviewing questionnaires, the researchers discovered something odd. Among the folks with respiratory ailments, there were very few fish-eaters. In fact, those who said they ate the least fish (two ounces or less each week) were 66 percent more likely to have bronchitis and 50 percent more likely to suffer with emphysema than those who averaged four servings.

"A link between a fishless diet and respiratory trouble isn't so farfetched, says Shahar. Although experts don't completely understand how cigarettes cause disease, most believe inhaled smoke damages the lungs by causing chronic irritation of the linings. Fish oil contains fatty acids that, in high doses, may reduce the inflammation. That could explain why lung disease is less common in Japan, for example. While many Japanese smoke, most eat heaps of seafood, too.

"According to Shahar, researchers soon will be giving fish oil to smokers to see if it eases damage to their lungs. But smokers shouldn't kid themselves. No matter what future studies find, it's clear a salmon fillet will never make up for the injury caused by cigarettes." (*Health*, 11-12/94)

lungs can sometimes be prevented by taking nutrients classified as antioxidants. These include vitamins A, C, E, B_1, B_5, B_6, the amino acid cysteine, zinc, selenium, and others.

Vitamins

Research conducted at the Delta Regional Primate Research Center at Tulane University seems to indicate that vitamin A helps protect the sensitive tissues in our lungs. The lungs use vitamin A to produce the necessary mucus cells to battle any foreign substances that might enter the lungs. Without adequate vitamin A, the lungs cannot produce mucus cells and the tissue becomes dry and hardened. According to the *Nutrition Almanac*, a therapeutic dosage of approximately 50,000 IU of vitamin A should be taken. Three to five thousand milligrams of vitamin C daily will also help provide basic protection of the healthy tissue in the respiratory passage.

Preventing Lung Disease

"A report in *Annals of the New York Academy of Sciences* showed the oxidation of lung tissue can be prevented with antioxidants, thereby helping to prevent lung disease. In both experimental animal and human experiments, the amount of antioxidants that offer protection was always in excess of the current recommended dietary allowance." (*Let's Live*, June 1995)

Since emphysema is a disease of the lungs, getting enough oxygen is of primary importance to its victims. Many experts agree that supplementing your diet with high doses of vitamin E will slow the destruction of your blood's ability to distribute oxygen. Durk Pearson and Sandy Shaw said in *Life Extension*, "High doses of E — in excess of 1,000 IU daily — frequently cause a dramatic improvement in skin appearance. This difference is sometimes noticeable in a few days, but a month is a more usual period over which to notice these results."

The *Nutrition Almanac* says vitamin E works to prevent the oxidation of vitamin A and recommends that emphysema patients take up to 1,600 IU per day.

Cigarette smoke contains another hazardous chemical called acetaldehyde. While experimenting with acetaldehyde, Dr. Herbert Sprince found that when large doses of the chemical were given to rats, 90 percent of them died. However, Pearson and Shaw indicate that when the very effective nutrient combination of vitamins B1 and C and cysteine were given to the rats with the same dose of acetaldehyde, none of the rats died. They recommend taking 1/2 to one gram of B_1, three to 10 grams of vitamin C, and one to three grams of cysteine (at least three times as much vitamin C as cysteine).

Another nutrient that is vital for normal respiration is copper. The body uses copper (and iron) for the synthesis of hemoglobin and in the production of elastin (the substance which makes our blood vessels, lungs, and skin flexible). According to the book *Amazing Medicines the Drug Companies Don't Want You to Discover!*, "Copper also combines to form enzymes that protect the body from oxidation damage. It is one of the most important blood antioxidants ... and contributes to the integrity of cell membranes, so essential to the limitation of the production of free radicals.... Copper deficiencies are thought to be responsible for lung damage from emphysema."

Copper supplementation should consist of two to three milligrams per day. Foods rich in copper include animal livers, seafood, nuts, fruits, and dried legumes.

Herbs

In addition to vitamin supplementation, emphysema sufferer's might try one of the following herbal treatments.

According to *Alternative Medicine: The Definitive Guide*, Dr. John A. Sherman of Portland, Oregon recommends a variety of herbal remedies: "Coltsfoot tea is effective in helping raise and eliminate mucus. Anise oil mixed with honey is very beneficial when taken before each meal. The active ingredients of thyme help to break up lung secretions and speed their elimination. Ephedra tea quiets bronchospasms. And mullein helps prevent infections and aids in excreting fluid from the lungs."

David L. Hoffman adds that combining specific herbs together can work very well. He said, "Relief from coughing may be expedited with a pleasant-tasting mixture of equal parts of coltsfoot, mullein, and licorice, taken three times a day. The flowers of these herbs, combined into an infusion, are not only effective, but taste delicious. A blend of marshmallow, mallow, coltsfoot, violet, mullein, and red poppy flowers in equal parts, taken three times a day, is another very 'pleasant' medicine. White horehound is also highly effective in battling coughing, but its unpleasant taste needs to be masked by combining it with licorice or anise seed."

Having emphysema can be a miserable experience for its victims, but taking a few steps in the right direction can make a world of difference. Hopefully these remedies are the guide you are looking for. And if you don't suffer from emphysema, please share this book with someone who does. We want to help as many people as we can.

[*Editor's Note: The reason few home remedy books offer suggestions for the home treatment of emphysema is that once the damage has been done to the lungs, it is almost impossible to reverse. However, we do know of a doctor-administered treatment that has achieved miraculous reversals. It is called intravenous hydrogen peroxide. If you would like more information about this treatment, please read Dr. William Campbell Douglass' book,* Hydrogen Peroxide: Medical Miracle *(Second Opinion Publishing, $12.95 plus $1.95 for shipping and handling, 800-728-2288). Or you can contact the International Oxidative Medicine Association (IOMA) at P.O. Box 891954, Oklahoma City, OK 73189 for a current list of doctors in your region that perform this therapy.*]

Chapter 8

Dealing with Hay Fever

Ah, springtime! It's such a glorious time of year, with gentle breezes, budding trees, blooming flowers, and ... ah ... aah ... aaachoo! Hay fever!

For 22 million Americans, springtime can be absolutely miserable. Uncontrollable sneezing that makes your lower jaw feel like it could pop off at any time. Not to mention the clogged nasal passages, runny nose, and watery eyes that add up to long days with no relief.

Hay fever has nothing to do with hay and it rarely produces a fever, but few conditions are as frustrating to treat. And allergy sufferers usually rely on over-the-counter (OTC) remedies that are often less than useful, including nasal sprays, decongestants, and antihistamines.

Some have found limited relief with the OTC drugs, but for many, the side effects can be miserable. Dr. Charles Banov, an allergist and past president of the American College of Allergy and Immunology, says that if they're used for more than three days, nasal sprays can actually increase congestion: "What happens is, you actually get a change in nose tissue and you require more and more of the medicine for the tissue to shrink. Finally, you have to use so much and spray it so often to get the effects that the nose drops act as an irritant." This increased dosage can also lead to addiction.

In addition, using decongestants and antihistamines can cause high blood pressure, insomnia, irritability, and rebound congestion.

But there are several ways that you can turn nature against itself to relieve the frustrating symptoms of hay fever. An old folk tale says that growing somewhere near the plant causing your troubles is another plant that will cure your troubles. That tale may or may not be true, but

---

A Honey of a Cure

You've heard of honey's antibacterial properties, but did you know that it's also a great immune system booster especially for hay fever? Eating raw, unprocessed, and unheated honey from *your area* will greatly aid your battle against these dreaded allergies. The daily ingestion of honey (one to three teaspoons a day, taken with meals) acts as a kind of vaccination for pollen allergies. When bees make honey, tiny particles of your local pollen are part of its composition and eating it allows your immune system to build up a resistance against the pollen. Taken over a long period of time (usually more than a year), many people have found that this remedy works quite well. Check with a local beekeeper and find honey that was made while the offending pollens were around. (*Joy of Health*, 2/95)

we do know that there are herbs that can help stabilize the immune system; others that reduce inflammation of mucous membranes; and some herbs even inhibit the cells that produce and release histamines (the chemical that causes tissue redness and swelling as well as increased mucous production).

An Interesting Fact About Hay Fever

A recent study of 17,400 children found that the more siblings a child has, the less likely he is to contract hay fever. Based on his observations, David Strachan, a British epidemiologist, theorizes that children born into big families have stronger immune systems because of their exposure to a large number of childhood diseases.

Strachan's research may help explain why hay fever is a modern phenomenon. With the shift from an agrarian society to an industrial society, the average number of children born to each family has dropped significantly. Also, life on the farm is much dirtier than life in the industrial age, giving the immune system a more vigorous workout. As a result, an improved standard of living and better hygiene may have made us more vulnerable than our forbearers to pollen. (*Edell Health Letter*, 4/90)

Taking Precautions, Not Drugs

The first step is boosting your immune system. To do this, start preparing your body for allergy season four to six weeks before it hits. Drink six to 12 glasses of water a day (the more you weigh, the more you need to drink). You should be drinking this much water anyway, but it's especially important during allergy season. We reported on a few of the values of water in the other chapters of this book, so you already know that dehydration severely affects the immune system. But what most people don't realize is that water helps lower the concentration of histamines in the cells.

Dr. Earl Mindell recommends boosting your immune system by taking "a regimen of two weeks of the herb echinacea followed by two weeks of the herb astragalus. Take two capsules, three times daily.... Take each herb for two weeks on, then two weeks off so your body stays sensitive to them." (*Joy of Health*, 2/95) Both herbs are available at your local health food store.

Mindell also recommends eating plenty of garlic, yogurt, and shiitake and Reishi mushrooms. "Garlic is a potent antioxidant," he says, "keeping cells healthy, intact, and running smoothly." Eating one to two cups of yogurt each day will significantly reduce your allergy symptoms and eating one or two mushrooms a week is a great way to strengthen your immune system.

Jane Guiltinan, N.D., the chief medical officer at the Natural Health Clinic at Bastyr College, a naturopathic college in Seattle, Washington, "recommends taking two or three tablespoons daily of black currant oil, flaxseed oil, or evening primrose oil during the hay-fever season as a preventive measure." These essential fatty acids will help reduce your body's production of the inflammatory agents that swell mucous membranes. (*Vegetarian Times*, 8/93)

Drug-Free Relief

Now that we've taken a few steps to boost your immune system, let's look at several drug-free ways to reduce the misery of hay-fever.

If you were to visit an herbalist or a naturopath, the list of herbs they could tell you to use for allergies would be full of effective remedies. But due to space, we'll limit our discussion to a few that deserve special mention.

According to the *Vegetarian Times*, "Both licorice root and Siberian ginseng support the adrenal glands, which produce a hormone called cortisol, an anti-inflammatory agent that reduces swelling of mucous membranes. You can make licorice or ginseng tea by steeping a teaspoon of chopped-up root in a cup of simmering water for 15 minutes; strain and drink several cups per day. (People with high blood pressure should avoid these herbs, however, because they can exacerbate hypertension; also, don't take them month after month without professional supervision.)"

Freeze-Dried Nettles

Probably the most helpful herb for hay fever is freeze-dried stinging nettle. In 1982, two physicians "showed that the active components of the stinging hairs, acetylcholine, serotonin, and histamine, normally destroyed in the drying process, had been preserved." (*East West Natural Health*, 3-4/92)

In 1990, *Planta Medica* published the randomized, double-blind study. In this study, half of the experimental group took two 300-mg capsules of nettle at the onset of symptoms and half received a placebo. Fifty-eight percent of the subjects in the experimental group rated nettle as moderately to highly effective in relieving hay-fever symptoms. Forty-eight percent said nettle was as effective, if not more so, than the drugs they had previously used.

Don't expect nettles to work in every case, because they aren't a miracle cure. Some people have found that dairy products prohibit the nettles from working. If they don't work for you, cut all dairy products out of your diet and try them again. To use nettle throughout the season, take two or three capsules twice a day. Freeze-dried nettle capsules can be found in your local health food store.

More Herbs Worth Mentioning

Corrine Martin, a certified herbalist, has found several herbs that consistently work against hay-fever symptoms. All of them are safe to use, except for a few that are discouraged during pregnancy. Because they are safe, you can choose the ones that address your specific symptoms and combined their tinctures to make a remedy that's more personalized. Try one or more of the following, you might be pleasantly surprised.

"Eyebright: The aerial parts (any part of the plant above ground) of this tiny plant are both astringent and anti-inflammatory, and decrease the hypersensitive response of the mucous membranes in the eyes, nose, throat, and ears. In other words, this herb is the perfect remedy for hay-fever sufferers.... While it grows wild in

Making a Tincture

Many of the remedies mentioned in this chapter are best taken in a tincture. A tincture is similar to a tea except that it's made with alcohol or vinegar instead of water. Because of this difference, tinctures are more concentrated than teas and require only a few drops to a tablespoonful for each dosage. To make a tincture:

1. Cut the plant parts into small pieces and pack it in a large jar with a screw-top lid.

2. Cover the herb with brandy, vodka, or gin (if you use cider vinegar instead of alcohol, double the recommended dosages). If the herb floats to the top of the jar, place a clean stone on top of it to keep it immersed.

3. Seal the jar and store it in a dark, cool, dry spot for two weeks, shaking it occasionally.

4. At the end of the two weeks, strain off the liquid through coffee filters or several layers of cheese cloth into another clean, dark bottle for storage. Some herbalists recommend that you send the herb through a wine press to squeeze out all the juice.

5. Make sure you label the storage jar with the name of the herb and the date. You might also want to specify whether it was prepared in alcohol or vinegar. Alcohol preparations will last almost indefinitely, but herbs prepared in vinegar will last for only two to three years.

some eastern and northeastern states, including Maine, New Hampshire, Massachusetts, and New York, you can purchase preparations of eyebright in most herb or health food stores. Dosage: Take as tea (one teaspoon of dried plant per one cup of boiling water) or in tincture form (approximately 30 drops), four to six times daily.

"Golden Seal: The bitter, yellow root of this wild flower has antibiotic properties and is useful in preventing secondary infection in hay fever, sinusitis, or chest congestion. It is also anti-inflammatory to the mucous membranes, and helps reduce and soothe swollen, irritated tissues. Therefore, golden seal is helpful in all types of airborne allergy responses.... It is probably best purchased from organic growers. (Caution: Golden seal may stimulate mild uterine contractions, so it is unsafe to ingest during pregnancy.) Dosage: Take as tincture (30 drops) or as tea (use one teaspoon per one cup water; and be warned that it tastes extremely bitter), four to six times daily.

"Mullein: The fuzzy leaves of the common biennial weed are expectorant, decongestant, and mildly sedative to respiratory mucous membranes. Mullein calms inflamed lung tissue and enhances moistening of the tiny air sacs in the lungs.... Dosage: Take as tea (one tablespoon dried herb per one cup boiling water) or tincture (30 to 60 drops), four to six times daily....

"Violet: The leaves and blossoms of this common plant are both an expectorant and decongestant, and soothe irritated mucous membranes of the lungs. Violets also act as a lymphatic-system stimulant, helping to relieve a buildup of toxins in the body.... The violet can be harvested in the wild or purchased from a local plant nursery and transplanted into flower beds where it will flourish. Dosage: Take as tea (one tablespoon per one cup water) or take in tincture form (30 to 60 drops), four to six times daily....

"One of my favorite remedies for hay fever is a mixture of tinctures of echinacea, golden seal, eyebright, stinging nettles, and Siberian ginseng. People I've offered it to swear by it and call every allergy season for more." (*Mother Earth News*, 3-4/93)

Final Thoughts

As you can see, there are many herbs that have been proven to work against pollen allergies — and we've just mentioned a few. But there are other things you need to be considering as spring approaches. The healthier you

---

Airing Out Allergies

"Researchers in Australia have found that airing removable rugs outside on a sunny day may be one of the best ways to help prevent allergies. Placing the rugs upside down, for four hours, in the hot sun, effectively killed 100 percent of the dust mites and their eggs.

"Dust mites are one of the main household culprits triggering asthma attacks, allergic reactions, and sinus problems. (For rugs and furnishings that can't be removed, treating them with tannic acid seems to be the most effective method of eliminating mites.)" (*Alternatives*, October 1994)

are, the better your body can battle the invading allergens. If you're stressed, exhausted, or just generally run-down, you've placed a heavy burden on your immune system. Make sure you're getting plenty of rest and exercise and eating a healthy diet with plenty of protein. These are essential to good health.

Also, check your home for possible allergen "traps." Carpets, rugs, and draperies are filled with dust mites during this time of year. So make sure you take special precautions to deal with these annoying creatures.

Chapter 9

Bronchitis and Sinusitis

One of our subscribers recently sent us a most fascinating health book. The 1,680-page tome is simply called *The National Dispensatory*. What could possibly be so fascinating about *The National Dispensatory*? For one thing, this particular one was published in 1880.

Many of the potions this massive book mentions are now obsolete, but *The National Dispensatory* of 1880 contains many enchanting medical secrets that I'd like to share with you.

Take for instance the unusual (and some not-so-unusual) treatments it lists for bronchitis. Opening up to the index, we find close to 200 remedies for bronchitis, but the ones listed below are still known as effective bronchitis fighters. Try them and see.

Anise

"Anise is an aromatic stimulant and carminative, and its oil and infusion are habitually employed to relieve flatulent colic.... It has been imagined to have some special influence upon the bronchial tubes, modifying their secretions and promoting expectoration." It's effectiveness isn't just imagined anymore. According to modern studies, anise loosens bronchial secretions making them easier to cough up.

To make an infusion, gently crush one teaspoon of anise seeds per cup of boiling water and steep for 10 to 20 minutes. Strain and drink up to three cups per day. If being used to treat colic in infants, dilute the infusion.

Eucalyptus

"Not being an irritant, eucalyptus may be liberally used ... in all cases of ulcer of the stomach or bowels, in septicemia, and fetid bronchitis.... It has been inhaled with great advantage in cases of fetid bronchitis." You may have noticed eucalyptus in many of your throat lozenges because of its ability to clear mucus from the lungs. Steeping a handful of fresh or dried leaves in a quart of water for 20 minutes makes a simple infusion. Drink two cups daily.

Grindelia

"Grindelia has a persistent acrid and bitter taste, and excites the secretion of saliva. It is said to reduce the respiration rate, to stimulate the brain and the spinal cord, and subsequently to produce a tendency to repose or sleep, with impaired power of the legs.... The herb of this plant is reported to be useful in whooping cough and bronchitis, and of singular efficacy in asthma. We have been informed of several cases occurring in aged persons, in which half a teaspoonful of the fluid extract afforded almost instantaneous relief.... The dose for a child two years old is stated to be 10 drops every two hours of the fluid extract."

Mix 15 grams in 500 ml of water for an infusion. For adults, take up to five ml a day in doses of one-two ml.

Horehound

"Anciently regarded as a general stimulant, expectorant, deobstruent, carminative, and local anodyne, horehound continues to be employed as a stomach tonic in dyspepsia, and in chronic bronchitis to restrain secretion.... An infusion, made with an ounce of horehound in a pint of hot water, may be given in doses of a wineglassful."

Vitamin C Helps Elderly Bronchitis and Pneumonia Patients

"In a double-blind trial, 57 elderly hospital patients with bronchitis or bronchopneumonia were randomly assigned to 200 mg vitamin C or placebo for four weeks. Signs and symptoms were significantly reduced in the vitamin C group, total respiratory clinical scores dropping 48 percent in the vitamin C group compared with 31 percent in the control group." (*Clinical Nutrition Update*, December 1994)

Vitamin C and Upper Respiratory Infections

"Marathon runners frequently get upper respiratory infections during the two-week period following a race, although the reasons for this are not well-understood. But now these athletes may escape such infections entirely, or at least lessen their severity. In a study by scientists at the University of the Witwatersrand in Johannesburg, South Africa, researchers gave marathon runners either a placebo (an inactive substance) or put them on a supplementation regime consisting of 600 mg of vitamin C per day.

"During the 14 days after the race, 65 percent of the placebo group developed symptoms of upper respiratory disease, while only 33 percent of the vitamin-C supplemented group reported such symptoms. Also, in the group that received vitamin C, those who did get upper respiratory infections reported significantly less severe symptoms and significantly shorter duration of symptoms than did those in the placebo group.

"The researchers say the study provides evidence that vitamin C supplementation may enhance resistance to the upper respiratory infections commonly suffered by marathon runners in the post-race period." (*Health Line*, 11-12/95)

Jujube

"In the native countries of the jujube, its fruit is ranked with figs and raisins and other more or less saccharine and acidulous fruits, which are used in tisanes (infusions) for acute irritations of the throat and air passages, much as in this country we employ the syrup and jelly of currants, blackberries, etc."

Magnolia

"The bark of the several medicinal species of magnolia ... has been used in hot decoction to produce diaphoresis in fevers, bronchial catarrhs, rheumatism, and gout, and in cold decoction or tincture as a tonic. The tree is said to render clear the waters near which it grows, and to prevent malarial affections.... The dose of the recently dried bark in powder is stated to be from 30 to 60 grains, frequently repeated."

A Drug-Free Treatment for Sinusitis

Sinusitis is an inflammation of the nasal passage due to an infection of the air-filled cavities that surround the nasal passage. This aggravation often follows the common cold or hay fever and usually makes breathing very difficult, unpleasant, and painful.

Most doctors will employ a series of antihistamines, decongestants, and antibiotics to deal with the infection.

When these don't work, they resort to surgery, thinking it's the only way to relieve the symptoms.

Unfortunately, symptoms are all surgery can address. It doesn't deal with the underlying cause of the infection. As a result, you can often treat sinusitis at home more effectively than your doctor can. Here's how:

Watch That Diet

Richard Barrett, N.D., associate academic dean of the National College of Naturopathic Medicine in Portland, Oregon, says treatment should begin with a water fast for a day or two to allow the body to work on fighting the infection and not on digesting food. Or you can eat a very light diet that avoids all concentrated sugars and consists mainly of fruits and vegetable broth.

Gingerly Treat Upper Respiratory Infections

Dr. Alan R. Gaby reported in the June 1995 issue of *Nutrition & Healing* that ginger tea is an effective "treatment for sore throats, laryngitis, and other symptoms associated with upper respiratory tract infections. Ginger tea can be prepared by peeling off the thin brown coating, dicing about four inches of the root, and simmering for 45 minutes in a quart-and-a-half of water. The tea may be sipped throughout the day as needed."

Next, Dr. Barrett advises the following regimen of nutritional supplementation (as published in *Alternative Medicine*):

* **Vitamin A:** 50,000 IUs per day for one week only, or beta carotene: 200,000 IUs per day.
* **Vitamin C:** One gram per hour to bowel tolerance.
* **Vitamin E:** 400 IUs per day.
* **Zinc:** 50 mg per day.

If you suffer from chronic sinusitis, Dr. Barrett recommends you add 200 mcg of selenium, 500 mg of N-acetyl cysteine, and one to two grams of bioflavonoids per day.

Homeopathy and Herbs

Dr. H.C.A. Vogel, author of *The Nature Doctor*, says, "Onion poultices, while perhaps not very pleasant, are simple and effective. Chop an onion finely, place it between two pieces of gauze and bind it on the neck before retiring, leaving it overnight. The two homeopathic remedies Hepar sulph. 4x and Cinnabaris 4x will help eliminate the pus and heal the affected part.... For a chronic case, or when the trouble originated with a cold, hot compresses and baths always soothe and alleviate the pain."

The Japanese use a spoonful of horseradish and the Mexicans are served a healthy dose of red-hot chili peppers (Africans use cayenne pepper) to ease sinusitis troubles.

In England, people with sinus infections, as well as coughs and bronchitis, make an interesting concoction using cabbage and honey. According to *Natural Health Secrets* (Shot Tower Books, 1994), "Cabbage syrup is made by liquefying a red cabbage in the blender. The juice is strained and weighed, and half its weight in honey is added. The mixture is simmered over a low heat until syrupy. Several doses of two teaspoonfuls each can be taken in quick succession. Cabbage is an excellent source of vitamin C, and the honey soothes the throat." Honey is also an excellent infection fighter.

Chapter 10

Questions and Answers

Bronchitis

Q. My family lives in the Puget Sound area of Washington. Due to the rainy conditions of this area we have a terrible time with bronchitis. Is there anything we can do to lessen our chances of getting bronchitis?

A. Residents of Britain live in a very wet climate and are also prone to suffer from bronchitis. So do the people around the Mediterranean, but the number of people there who actually contract the disease is much lower than in Britain. Why? Dr. Irwin Ziment of the Los Angeles County-Olive View Medical Center in Van Nuys, California, says that one reason the difference may exist is due to the high levels of garlic consumption. In the Mediterranean region, food is spiced more heavily with garlic than in Britain. Dr. Ziment, as reported in the *Journal of the American Medical Association*, believes that garlic may prevent bronchitis by loosening the mucus in the bronchi, and thus stopping its buildup.

If you should come down with a bad case of bronchitis, don't count on getting help from the drug store. There is no scientific evidence that expectorants, or any other drug for that matter, dry up mucus. If you are coughing up sputum, stay away from cough syrups. A productive cough is your body's way of ridding itself of unwanted mucus in the lungs — an action you don't want to suppress. Eating a healthy amount of garlic and getting plenty of rest in a warm bed is your best treatment for bronchitis.

Asthma

Q. I have a 14-year-old daughter who has been troubled by asthma nearly all her life. One doctor has told us that she would probably outgrow it. The fact is, she hasn't improved at all and now seems to be getting worse. She takes a ventolin inhaler and recently this is bringing her less and less relief. I hope you can help us with some effective recommendations.

A. New research from the University of Arizona is indicating that all cases of asthma are caused by allergies. Dr. Benjamin Burrows reported in the *New England Journal of Medicine* (320,5:271) that, "These findings challenge the concept that there are basic differences between so-called allergic (extrinsic) and nonallergic (intrinsic) forms of asthma."

The study consisted of 2,600 volunteers with asthma or allergic rhinitis and concluded that the prevalence of asthma was directly related to the level of the serum immunoglobulin (IgE) in the body. "And no asthma was present in the 177 subjects with the lowest IgE levels for their age and sex," the researchers reported.

According to the *Book of Proven Home Remedies and Natural Healing Secrets*, "IgE is the antibody that causes immune system response in the body. When your body has an allergic reaction — in other words, when your immune system overreacts to a stimulus — you get excessive amounts of the antibody IgE in your body."

The study showed that asthma is caused by some type of IgE-related action and therefore has an allergic basis. And other studies suggest that asthma in children might be caused by an allergy to house-dust mites — microscopic spider-like creatures that cling to specks of dust.

The author of this study, Dr. Richard Sporik, said, "Over the past 30 years, many of the changes we have made in our houses — such as increased temperatures and the use of fitted carpets, tighter insulation, and detergents effective in cool water — have improved the conditions needed for dust mites to grow."

There are several things you can do to rid your home of dust mites. For starters, choose washable bedding, not wool or down blankets, and wash it weekly in hot water. It is also suggested that you remove any heavy curtains, Venetian blinds, and carpet. However, before doing so, you might want to try a spray that contains tannic acid, a compound found in oak bark, coffee, and tea. The acid is designed to alter house dust, pollen, and dust-mite debris so that the body no longer has an allergic reaction to them. You can find tannic acid sprays in most pet stores. Be sure to follow the manufacturer's directions.

Allergies

Q. I really enjoyed your article on hay fever (page 79) and have tried several of the remedies you recommended. I found that drinking more water really helped and the freeze-dried nettles worked quite well, too, but neither completely cured my problem. I was wondering if you had any other treatments that could put me over the top?

A. Actually, there are several things you can do to get "over the top." But due to space, I'll only address a few. The first thing you need to do is increase your intake of vitamin C to two to five grams, three times per day with meals (that's six to 15 grams a day). It is recommended that you start with smaller doses and work your way up to the larger doses. If it causes diarrhea, reduce the dosage.

Next, Dr. Marcus Laux suggests that you "take bioflavonoids. I recommend a product called HMC from Thorne Research, which contains a special form of the bioflavonoid hesperidin. Take one to two capsules (250 mg each), three times per day with meals. (It's sold only through health practitioners. To find a practitioner near you who stocks it, call 800-228-1966.) This very absorbable bioflavonoid family member works like an antihistamine, only without side effects, other than an occasional dry nasal passage. Simply reduce the dosage until it normalizes if this happens. Another great source of bioflavonoids is Turmeric/Catechu Supreme from Gaia Herbs. This one you'll find in health food stores. Take as directed."

Since the freeze-dried nettles did you some good, you might try a special herbal combination also recommended by Dr. Laux: "Eyebright/Nettles Combination from Herb Pharm Co., or Eyebright/ Bayberry Supreme from Gaia Herbs, one dropperful, three times per day between meals. Both contain traditional botanical medicines for allergy relief and immune support. You'll find them in health food stores." (*Naturally Well*, 4/95)

Section 3

Heart Problems

Chapter 11

Preventing and Treating Heart Disease

"What a beautiful tee shot," Lester thought to himself. "Right down the middle of the fairway."

The drive almost caught him off guard. A rusty front nine and a few rough holes on the back nine made it a welcome (if not surprising) shot. It was the first time all day Lester wished there was someone around to see him play.

The course wasn't too busy. Lester had retired from his engineering job several months before and was able to play while the rest of the world went to work.

He wasn't playing the best game of his life, but that didn't matter. The rainy spring weather had kept him off the course for several weeks, so it was nice just to be outside and playing again.

Tragically, the ball never moved from the center of the fairway.

Lester liked to walk the golf course to get some exercise, and while walking from the tee box to the ball, he suffered a massive heart attack. The golfers in the next group found him and called the paramedics. But it was too late.

The First Symptom

It's not the kind of story we like to read, but Lester's story is one we see all too often. That's because heart disease is still the number one killer of Americans, despite the substantial work science has done to defeat it.

Heart Disease and Antioxidants

The results of a new study indicate that antioxidants are some of the best supplements you can take to protect yourself from heart disease.

"In this study, 5,133 Finnish men and women — ages 30 to 69 years — who were free from heart diseases were evaluated to find a relationship between antioxidants and heart disease. Vitamins C, E, and carotene were included in the subjects' diets.

"In the 14-year, follow-up study, 244 cases of fatal coronary heart disease occurred. Results showed there was an inverse relationship between the amount of vitamin E ingested and the death rate for heart disease in both men and women. Women showed a similar inverse relationship to coronary heart disease when vitamin C and carotenoids (from vegetables and fruits) were studied.

"Taking antioxidants is greatly enhanced by eating dark green, yellow, and red fruits and vegetables. Therefore, people should eat their veggies and take antioxidant supplements for healthier hearts." (*Let's Live*, February 1995)

For many people, the first symptom of heart disease is a heart attack. That's not the way you want to learn about this problem. So it's extremely important to understand why people get heart disease and then take the proper steps to avoid it.

Vitamin C and Good Cholesterol

"Until now, the only factor known to raise levels of high-density lipoprotein (HDL), the 'good cholesterol' that helps transport low-density lipoprotein (LDL, the 'bad cholesterol') out of the body, has been exercise. But a new study provides compelling evidence that HDL cholesterol rises in step with blood levels of vitamin C.

"Paul Jacques, Sc.D., and his coworkers at Tufts University's Human Nutrition Research center on Aging found that women's HDL peaked when vitamin C in the blood reached one milligram per deciliter. For men, the HDL continued to rise in parallel with vitamin C, while the LDL or 'bad' cholesterol dropped significantly.

"According to Jacques, a study involving elderly men and women found that men's blood levels of vitamin C reached one milligram per deciliter when they had consumed about 150 mg of vitamin C; women needed about 90 mg — the amount in six ounces of orange juice — to reach the same level. The best bet for both men and women is eating several helpings daily of foods rich in vitamin C." (*Natural Health*, 1-2/95)

Because heart disease is such a major problem in this country, you may be thinking that modern medicine knows the most effective ways to treat it. But, as is the case so often, modern medicine is now confirming what those in the alternative-health field have known for years: You can prevent and treat many cases of heart disease at home.

No, we don't want you to stay away from your doctor on this one, but most of the things we will be discussing can be done in addition to your doctor's treatments. Be sure to check out the Editor's Note on page 140 that tells you what doctor-administered treatment you need, in addition to home treatment.

The Studies Prove It

Nutritional supplementation for the prevention of heart disease has been scoffed at for years by the medical establishment. But doctors are slowly waking up to the reality that studies supporting the use of supplements have been filling the medical literature for some time.

In 1993, the *New England Journal of Medicine* published the results of a study from Harvard Medical School and Brigham and Women's Hospital in Boston. The study followed 87,245 nurses for eight years and found that many women can reduce their risk for heart disease by 40 percent. How? Simply by taking vitamin E supplements for two years or more.

Elizabeth Sommer, M.A., R.D., said in the June 1993 issue of the *Nutrition Report*, "The Harvard study is by no means a lone wolf. It merely adds more credibility to what we already know — antioxidants, in amounts greater than usually consumed in the diet, are good for you."

Antioxidants to the Rescue

You may have noticed that I didn't come right out and recommend a low-cholesterol diet to prevent heart disease. That's because cholesterol is not the cause of heart disease! A high cholesterol count is a symptom, not a disease, and we want to treat the problem.

Chemist and medical researcher David R. Schryer says that our bodies require the presence of adequate concentrations of antioxidants in order to prevent destructive oxidation of our cells, and their constituent parts, by free radicals.

What most people don't realize is that the process of neutralizing free radicals causes the antioxidants to be used up. Because of this, the body requires much larger quantities of antioxidants than most other nutrients.

When America was largely an agrarian society, we acquired most of the vitamins we needed from the foods we grew and raised. Unfortunately, today's Americans don't eat the same foods. Instead, we eat processed food and other foods that are low in antioxidants. That means that free radicals can do more damage if we don't have some antioxidant supplementation.

According to Schryer, "Statistics indicate that less than 10 percent of Americans eat a healthy diet, with several servings of fruits and vegetables each day. Furthermore, of the relatively few fruits and vegetables which most of us eat, many are either picked green and 'ripened' in transit or highly processed. Therefore, most people are not ingesting adequate quantities of the major antioxidants, especially vitamin C. Consequently, the cells and organs of many people have undergone — and are still undergoing — continuous destructive assault by free radicals.

"Our bodies do not accept continuous assault by metabolically generated free radicals — combined with inadequate nutrient intake — without a fight. If we do not provide our bodies with enough of the dietary antioxidants which they need, they fall back upon an antioxidant which they can manufacture themselves: cholesterol."

That's right. Cholesterol is an antioxidant. And your body produces it as a last-ditch effort to correct a deficiency. This also explains why the cholesterol levels of people who go on low-cholesterol diets refuse to lower. It's not the cholesterol in your diet that is causing the elevated levels, it's the lack of antioxidants in your diet.

What Type and How Much?

In order for antioxidant supplementation to work effectively against heart disease, we must change our mind-set in regards to how we take vitamins. We must have a proactive attitude. Instead of asking how much is enough, we must ask how much is too much and then stay below that level. The truth is, our bodies require rather large amounts of vitamins C and E, beta carotene, and Coenzyme Q10 (CoQ10) to effectively battle cell-destroying free radicals.

So how much of the various anti-oxidants do you need to take to prevent heart disease? As is the case with most medical conditions, every case is different. But what follows are general guidelines for taking antioxidants and other supplements that can be safely administered at home. If you wish to have a more personalized regimen,

Folic Acid Deficiency Linked to Strokes and Heart Attacks

In 1948, researchers began studying 5,209 residents of Framingham, Massachusetts in what is now "the longest-running and most productive heart disease research project ever. Virtually all identifiable heart risk factors stem from this study.... Only 1,400 of the original subjects are still living, but the study continues, now including a second generation of 5,000 who entered the program in 1971.

"A little more than three years ago, Tufts University researchers initiated a study of 1,000 elderly volunteers from the original Framingham group. The team wanted to see if there was a relationship between an amino acid called homocysteine and narrowing of the carotid artery caused by atherosclerotic plaque buildup....

"The Tufts University study showed that the Framingham subjects who were getting inadequate folic acid and B-vitamin in their diets — and who had low blood levels of folic acid, vitamin B_{12}, and vitamin B_6 — had carotid-artery stenosis, placing them at an increased risk for stroke. The study successfully linked an increased risk for vascular disease to elevated homocysteine levels and, more important, to low blood levels of folic acid, B_{12}, and B_6.

"In short, it appears that these vitamins can protect us from heart disease...." (*Saturday Evening Post*, May/June 1995)

you'll need to visit a nutritionally oriented doctor who can deal with your problem more specifically.

Vitamin C

You've heard how important this vitamin is and it's not a rumor. Our bodies require larger quantities of vitamin C than any other vitamin because the vitamin is involved in several important biochemical functions. Because of the number of roles vitamin C plays in our body, it is the vitamin most likely to be deficient. Researchers differ on how much vitamin C to recommend, but generally, you need at least 20 milligrams per day for every pound of body weight. That means a 150-pound person would need three grams (or 3,000 milligrams) per day. Some people have increased that dosage to 30 milligrams per pound of body weight. Large doses of vitamin C have not been found to be toxic, but if you take more than your body needs, you may get diarrhea.

Coenzyme Q10 (CoQ10)

CoQ10 is a fat-soluble vitamin and, like vitamin C, serves many important functions in the body, including energy production within the cell. It is a crucial vitamin for the prevention and treatment of heart disease. In fact, a CoQ10 deficiency has been found to be a major cause of congestive heart failure and cardiomyopathy. For preventive measures, it is good to follow a general rule of 0.5 mg of CoQ10 per pound of body weight, although

240 to 360 mg per day is not unusual for therapeutic treatment of heart disease.

Vitamin E

You've already seen the importance of vitamin E in preventing heart disease, so make sure you include it in your supplementation regimen. A daily dosage of 400 IU is recommended.

Magnesium

This is a mineral that is often ignored in the treatment of heart disease, but is one of the more critical supplements in your regimen. Along with a CoQ10 deficiency, people with heart disease frequently have a magnesium deficiency. The major sources for magnesium are dark-green leafy vegetables and "hard" water — both of which are not consumed in large quantities in the U.S. Adequate intake of magnesium (500 to 1,000 mg per day, in chelated form) contributes to a healthy heart and dramatically increases your survival chances if a heart attack does occur.

According to one study, "One hundred ninety-four patients hospitalized with an acute myocardial infarction (heart attack) were randomly assigned to receive an intravenous infusion of magnesium for 48 hours or a placebo infusion (glucose). Compared with the placebo, magnesium treatment significantly reduced the incidence of arrhythmias (heart-rhythm disturbances) and congestive heart failure and significantly improved the strength of the heart (measured as ejection fraction). The in-hospital death rate was 74 percent lower in the magnesium group than in the placebo group (four percent vs. 17 percent)." (*American Journal of Cardiology*, 1995;75:321-323; *Nutrition & Healing*, May 1995)

Beta Carotene

Take 10,000 to 25,000 IU every day.

Selenium

Taken in large doses, selenium can be very toxic. So make sure you take smaller doses of 100 to 200 mcg per day.

Researchers now agree that antioxidant levels are much more important than cholesterol levels in determining susceptibility to heart disease and heart attack. In fact, chemist David R. Schryer indicates that "adequate intakes of vitamin C and other antioxidants [and minerals] are capable of preventing atherosclerosis entirely in most people, even in people with moderately elevated cholesterol levels." And new evidence is showing that regular ingestion of these nutrients can actually reverse atherosclerosis that has already occurred (at least partially).

Now is the time to be thinking about your future health, not when it's too late.

Chapter 12

High Blood Pressure

In the world of cardiovascular diseases, high blood pressure has earned the nickname "the silent killer." It makes your risk of suffering a heart attack three times greater and your risk of stroke seven times greater than people with normal blood pressure — and it does this many times with very few symptoms.

Hypertension, the scientific name for high blood pressure, is "the most prevalent and most dangerous precipitating factor in the genesis of cardiovascular diseases, the leading cause of death in the United States and other industrialized countries," remarked one physician.

How prevalent is it? Some surveys indicate that over 60 million Americans have been diagnosed with this "disease."

But high blood pressure is not a disease, it's a symptom. It's the body's way of dealing with biochemical changes that a person can undergo for a variety of reasons, whether it be stress, a change in exercise habits, an increase in body weight, or some other factor.

Dr. George Meinig, author of *"NEW"trition*, gives this illustration: "If you run water through your garden hose, it exerts pressure on the hose walls in varying amounts, depending on whether flow is restricted at the end by a nozzle. Should the inner walls of the hose become clogged with dirt or ice, the same amount of flow would result in more pressure upon its walls. When arteries become clogged with cholesterol, calcium deposits, or lose their elasticity, increased pressure results."

It is important to understand that hypertension is a symptom and not a disease, because most modes of treatment given by modern medicine are designed to treat the pressure, not the source (or cause) of the pressure — a potentially dangerous proposition which can magnify the problem. For many Americans now on blood-pressure medication, the side effects can include lethargy, depression, nausea, impotence, or worse.

Going Nuts for the Heart

"Good news for walnut lovers! A study at California's Loma Linda University discovered that eating walnuts can lower levels of total cholesterol — and improve your ratio of good cholesterol to bad cholesterol. The amount of walnuts consumed in this study was seven times what the average American eats, but you won't need to eat that much to get some benefit.... Scientists believe their (walnuts) unsaturated fats are much better for you than the saturated fats in animal products. Another reason? Walnuts are a great natural source of vitamin E — and there aren't that many." (*One Step Ahead*, November 1994)

Is Alcohol Good?

"Another large study has highlighted the potential benefits of alcohol to health and longevity. But unlike previous studies, this one showed that only wine, not beer or hard liquor, was associated with a longer life and that its apparent protective effect was far greater than has been found elsewhere.

"The 12-year study, conducted among more than 13,000 men and women aged 30 to 70 who participated in the Copenhagen Heart Study, revealed that those who drank wine daily were much less likely to die during the study period than those who drank beer or liquor or no alcohol at all.

"The greatest benefit, a 49-percent reduction in mortality, was associated with drinking three to five glasses of wine a day, considerably more than the one to two drinks a day generally recommended by American health experts. Among the Danes who consumed one to two glasses of wine a day there was also a significant but lesser reduction in deaths.

"The Copenhagen study did not report causes of death other than cardiovascular disease." (*New York Times*, 5/5/95)

... Or Bad?

"Alcohol has many side effects that the average drinker does not always realize. A recent research study done in Great Britain shows that men who drink three or four beers daily are more prone to develop chronic nosebleeds, as compared to men who drink fewer than five beers per week. Alcohol is a known blood thinner and high levels can make blood less likely to clot in and around the nasal area." (*Let's Live*, 3/95; *British Medical Journal*, 9/94)

The Problems with Blood-Pressure Medication

Prescription medication does serve a purpose in treating hypertension, but many times these drugs make the problem worse or create other problems that can be devastating. That's why our goal is to augment, or in some instances replace, standard treatments. Of course, don't stop taking any blood-pressure medication without consulting your physician. A sudden cessation could be fatal.

Dr. Julian Whitaker, editor of *Health & Healing*, says, "The current use of drugs to lower high blood pressure, in my opinion, is insane. The thiazide diuretics (Hydrodiuril, Hydrochlorothiazide, Chlorthalidone) deplete your supplies of potassium and magnesium and elevate your triglyceride and cholesterol levels, thereby increasing the risk of a heart attack and cardiac arrhythmias. Indeed, studies have shown that vigorous treatment with these drugs actually increases the death rate.

"The beta blockers (Inderal, Tenormin, Lopressor) are notorious for causing impotence, fatigue, and depression.

"More recent entries to the high blood pressure drug sweepstakes are calcium channel blockers (Calan, Cardizem, Procardia). These also weaken the heart, and can damage the liver. Of course, magnesium, God's calcium channel blocker, essentially does the same thing as these drugs without side effects...."

So let's take a look at a number of ways we can lower our blood pressure naturally and, at the same time, maybe get away from these harmful medications.

The First Step

If you are diagnosed with high blood pressure, the first thing you'll hear your doctor say is that it's time to change your lifestyle. This would include increasing your physical activity and reducing your weight, sodium intake, and alcohol intake.

The participants of a recent study (*Journal of the American Medical Association*, 8/11/93) were given this advice about lifestyle changes and then were randomly assigned to six groups. According to the *Cardiovascular Wellness Newsletter* (9/93), "One group took no drugs in addition to their lifestyle changes, though they were given a placebo. The other five groups were each assigned a different blood-pressure medication. The results showed ... [that] nearly 60 percent of the participants who made lifestyle changes, but did not take a drug, had substantial blood-pressure reduction, and, by the end of the study, did not require the addition of a drug."

The study also recommended that if, "after six months of sustained effective lifestyle counseling, blood pressure remains at 140/90 or greater, consideration should be given to adding low-dose drug treatment." However, before agreeing to take drugs (or if you've been on drugs and would like to be free from them), you should try various natural treatments first. What follows are several remedies that have proven effective in many cases of high blood pressure. And best of all, every one of them is safe, simple, and natural.

Water

One of the most interesting and unusual treatments for high blood pressure comes as a result of the extensive research done by Dr. F. Batmanghelidj, a graduate of the prestigious St. Mary's Medical School of London University. According to *Amazing Medicines the Drug Companies Don't Want You to Discover*, Dr. Batmanghelidj found that "when your body has a water deficiency, it has to apply force to move water to the most needed area. That force or pressure is called hypertension. Therefore, high blood pressure is caused by dehydration.

"The doctor is at odds with the medical establishment because it prescribes diuretics to alleviate high blood pressure. Diuretics accelerate the movement of water out of your body."

Dr. Batmanghelidj goes against the establishment in another significant area as well. We said earlier that most doctors will recommend that a hypertension patient reduce his sodium intake. But Dr. Batmanghelidj claims that "salt is important because it keeps more water in the tissues." He says he has "hundreds of case histories of successfully lowering high blood pressure with water."

In addition to drinking more water, patients should avoid all caffeine, as it is a diuretic and causes the body to expel water more quickly. That includes chocolate, coffee, tea, and soft drinks.

The amount of water you need to drink to get the desired effect depends on your body size. Dr Batmanghelidj recommends "six glasses for small people; eight for the average-sized body; and 10-12 for the large or obese person."

Almost immediately you'll notice that you're urinating more than usual. Many people find that chronic constipation is relieved as well. The treatment is so easy, it would be foolish not to try it.

Potassium

In addition to drinking more water, you need to adjust your diet to include several minerals that have a well-deserved reputation for lowering high blood pressure. The first of these is potassium. Dr. Meinig recommends, "Fresh, raw fruits and vegetables which are high in potassium should be eaten more freely." These include bananas, potatoes, avocados, lima beans (cooked), oranges, and tomatoes.

There is no shortage of evidence linking higher potassium intake with lower blood pressure. One survey, reported in the *New Encyclopedia of Common Diseases*, compared 86 vegetarian Seventh Day Adventists to "86 nonvegetarian Mormons (both groups abstain from alcohol, nicotine, and caffeine)." While both groups had lower-than-average blood pressure, it was discovered that the Seventh Day Adventists (who consume large amounts of fruits and vegetables) had substantially lower blood pressure.

Many experts in the medical establishment argue that too much sodium causes blood pressure to rise. However, most of the studies involving the potassium/sodium ratio seem to indicate that the level of potassium consumed has a greater impact on high blood pressure than the amount of sodium.

In another study conducted at the London Hospital Medical College and reported in the *New Encyclopedia of Common Diseases*, "a group of 16 people with mild hypertension and a group with normal blood pressure received two different diets, each for a period of 12 weeks. During the first 12 weeks, both groups ate their normal diet, plus sodium tablets. During the second period, their normal diets were supplemented with potassium, and they were instructed to avoid excessively salty foods and not to add salt while cooking or at the table."

The researchers concluded that "the key factor in the startling drop in pressure during the high-potassium/low-sodium diet had been the increased potassium, since their regular diets included only a marginal rise in sodium but a much greater decline in potassium."

The Salt Connection

In fact, no studies have ever proven that salt causes high blood pressure. And, more importantly, severe salt restriction may actually be harmful for some people. At a recent American Heart Association meeting, blood pressure specialist Dr. Brent M. Egan told the audience that the blood pressure of men on a low-salt diet actually rose as much as five points.

How can this be true? Dr. William Campbell Douglass, editor of *Second Opinion*, asserts that the body changes, "by 'transmutation,' sodium into vital potassium." Therefore, a sodium deficiency could contribute to a potassium deficiency. But to do so, the body requires the right kind of salt. "I am referring, as you might have guessed, to sea salt," says Dr. Douglass. When the body is given natural sea salt, it is able to work this "bio-electronic miracle."

"Also, natural sea salt is an alkalinizer," Dr. Douglass continues. "An acidity of the body fluids is believed to be the cause of, or a contributor to, many illnesses. In severe trauma and infections, the body needs an emergency supply of potassium to repair the imbalance. The easiest way to provide this is to administer by mouth small doses of light grey Celtic sea salt dissolved in distilled water. A level teaspoonful in an eight-ounce glass of distilled water is enough. Taking this solution once a day for a maximum of four days can often work wonders. The potassium will be replenished quickly as the body 'transmutes' the sodium into potassium.

"People are often surprised at the dramatic improvement in health seen with this treatment. The acid/base level is quickly restored, allergies and skin conditions clear up, and there is a higher resistance to infections. This self-treatment is perfectly safe unless you have severe kidney disease or a pituitary abnormality."

Calcium and Magnesium

In order for cardiac and skeletal muscles to function properly, they must have a correct balance of calcium and magnesium. For the body to metabolize calcium it must have a sufficient supply of magnesium. For instance, a severe deficiency in magnesium will cause a dramatic drop in blood levels of calcium.

For over 50 years magnesium has been a mainstay in treating hypertension, because it induces muscle relaxation and is necessary for potassium function.

"In one study," says *Alternative Medicine*, "magnesium supplementation lowered blood pressure in 19 of 20 hypertensives, compared to zero of four in the control group. Dietary magnesium is found in nuts (almonds, cashews, pecans), rice, bananas, potatoes, wheat germ, kidney and lima beans, soy products, and molasses.... Magnesium helps to dilate arteries and ease the heart's pumping of blood."

Dr. Julian Whitaker, editor of *Health & Healing*, agrees: "Numerous studies have indicated that hard water, made hard primarily because of magnesium, prevents high blood pressure in those communities which have it. Furthermore, they have demonstrated that when given intravenously or by mouth, magnesium will often markedly lower blood pressure."

Dietary supplementation should consist of 150-600 mg of magnesium, but supplements by mouth may not be sufficient. "It's more effective to use magnesium glycinate, taurate, or aspartate, or even herbal magnesium such as red raspberry," contends *Alternative Medicine*.

In addition, "1,000 mg daily of calcium has been shown to lower blood pressure in hypertensives and young adults. Because many hypertensives have a lower daily calcium intake than people with normal blood pressure, calcium-rich foods, including nuts and leafy green vegetables, such as watercress and kale, should also supplement the diet."

While there is evidence that calcium and magnesium can help lower high blood pressure, Dr. Jose Villar believes that hypertensives should not expect miracles.

Villar states, "We think that calcium is best used as a preventive rather than as a treatment. After all, if you live a lifestyle for 20 to 25 years that facilitates high blood pressure, then starting on calcium isn't going to erase all that damage.

"In fact, trying to prevent increased blood pressure with calcium alone won't work if the rest of your life is crazy. But if, for example, you keep your weight down and limit the stress in your life, then adding more calcium may give you that extra margin of safety."

The Big Player

One of the most publicized natural treatments for high blood pressure is garlic. The herb's effect on hypertension has been studied extensively and people throughout the world have been treated with garlic, with a reported success rate of about 40 percent.

Lelord Kordel tells of three such instances in his book *Natural Folk Remedies*: "In the Indian state of Goa, natives carry small bottles of garlic juice, from which they take a nip whenever they feel the pressure starting to rise. Tribesmen of Medes, at the first sign of rising blood pressure, chew vigorously on bits of garlic until pressure returns to normal. The Menangkabaus of Indonesia do the same with grated garlic."

Whether the use of garlic to lower blood pressure works or not has been a hotly debated topic in the scientific community for years. Some people believe that if garlic does indeed lower the pressure, it is only temporary and therefore not of much use. However, Dr. William Campbell Douglass, editor of *Second Opinion*, disagrees with this assessment:

"I've seen some convincing reports that show garlic can reduce moderately high blood pressure. Early studies, particularly from Eastern Europe, indicated a drop of up to 30 mm/Hg in systolic pressure, and up to 20 mm/Hg decline in the diastolic pressure....

"More recent studies, however, show that a small amount of garlic, taken over time, will lower blood pressure by almost 10 percent. It takes several weeks for this drop to occur, but occur it does....

"A 1993 study reported in *Pharmacotherapy* (July-August 1993) used 2400 mg per day of 'a popular garlic preparation' on nine patients with high blood pressure. Patients were tested five hours after the dose and were found to have 'a significantly lower diastolic blood pressure.' This effect lasted from five to 14 hours after the dose of garlic was taken.

"More studies are needed before I could suggest using garlic alone to lower blood pressure.... Adding a garlic supplement to your daily routine is an additional way to lower pressure while offering your heart the anti-clotting protection that aspirin provides, *but without potentially harmful side effects.*

"A German doctor recently reported, rather plaintively, that every older person he knew was taking an herbal preparation of garlic."

Dr. F.G. Piotrowski, a member of the medical faculty at the University of Geneva, recommends that doctors make garlic capsules a part of their standard treatment of high blood pressure.

In an experiment, Dr. Piotrowski treated 100 hypertension patients with garlic oil. In three to five days the patients were relieved of their symptoms and within a week their blood pressure dropped an average of two centimeters.

Celery

If you think those numbers are impressive, wait until you hear about the results researchers are having with celery. That's right, celery.

Some scientists, including Dr. William J. Elliott, a pharmacologist at the University of Chicago's Pritzker School of Medicine, say that the stringy European herb has been a folk remedy for high blood pressure since 200 B.C.

According to Jean Carper, author of *Food: Your Miracle Medicine*, "Dr. Elliott became intrigued when Vietnamese graduate student Quang T. Le mentioned that his father's high blood pressure had been successfully treated by a traditional Asian doctor who prescribed celery. After Minh Le, 62-years old, ate two stalks of celery every day for a week, his blood pressure dropped from a high of 158/96 to a normal 118/82."

When Dr. Elliott fed a celery extract to laboratory rats with normal blood pressure for a couple of weeks, their blood pressure fell an average 12 to 14 percent. The doses were equivalent to four stalks of celery a day.

You may be wondering if other vegetables would work just as well as celery. After all, isn't celery part of the carrot family? According to Dr. Elliott, celery's effects on high blood pressure appear to be unique. "The active blood-pressure lowering compound is found in rather high concentrations in celery," he says, "and not in many other vegetables."

Dr. Elliott's research indicates that celery may work best for stress-related hypertension, which includes approximately half of all Americans with high blood pressure.

The interesting fact about celery is its sodium content, which is extremely high for a vegetable. Earlier we discussed the controversy that is stirring over dietary sodium and hypertension. With sodium-rich celery being such an effective blood-pressure-lowering agent, the lines of truth have become even more muddled.

Dr. Bernard Jensen, author of *Foods That Heal*, gives this food for thought: "Celery is generally known as a sodium food, and sodium is what we call the youth maintainer in the body. Sodium helps keep us young and active, and the muscles limber and pliable. Whenever there is a stiffness in the joints and creaking or cracking in the knees, we know we are lacking in sodium. Sodium is the one element that most people lack.

"When the tissues, joints, and arteries get hard, there is too much calcium in the body, and a softer element is needed. The element that counteracts calcium best is sodium. It helps keep calcium in solution."

Of course, you can always get too much of any good thing. But sodium that comes from your salt shaker and from natural foods is not something that you need to be concerned about. The *Journal of the American College of Nutrition* reported in August 1991 that nearly 80 percent of the salt Americans eat is added to their diet during food processing — not cooking. Only 11.3 percent of your salt intake is from cooking and table salt. This means you need to stop eating *all* processed foods to eliminate the sodium problem in your diet.

Celery also helps lower your blood pressure in one other way. Many people suffer from hypertension because of problems in their digestive tract. For this, Dr. Jensen recommends that "celery should be eaten often, because it is one of the best foods for keeping the body well. It neutralizes acids and is a good blood cleanser.... Sodium is one of the chemical elements needed so much in the walls of the stomach and in the intestinal tract. Celery is particularly good for these parts of the body." It will help that chronic constipation, as well.

To get the desired results, simply eat two to four stalks of celery every day. Many times this will only need to be continued for a few weeks. And don't peel the strings — they're great for the digestive system.

Cayenne Pepper

Another herb that's good for the digestive tract and for hypertension is cayenne pepper. The people of Mexico have fewer heart attacks than we do in this country and, as research has shown, one of the main reasons is because of the fiery chili peppers they eat.

In his book *Left for Dead*, Richard Quinn gives living proof of the pepper's ability to protect the circulatory system. In the book, he tells of the day he suffered a heart attack and the subsequent bypass surgery. After the surgery didn't "make me good as new," his doctor explained that there was nothing left to do. Modern medicine had done all it could.

Quinn didn't give up hope. A friend had told him to take some cayenne pepper capsules, which he did. The next morning, he felt like a new man. He's taken the capsules every day for 13 years and Quinn is still alive and healthy without a hint of any heart problems.

But Quinn isn't the only one who has been helped by cayenne pepper. This herb is renowned for its ability to regulate blood flow and strengthen the heartbeat and metabolic rate. And, much like garlic, cayenne helps prevent platelets from sticking together and forming dangerous blood clots.

Mannfried Pahlow, author of *Healing Plants*, says using hearty seasonings "often intensifies the progress of almost all vital processes, which results in increased vitality. If you want an all-around feeling of well-being, frequently add spicy seasonings like ... cayenne pepper ... to your foods."

The following testimonial in *Natural Home Remedies* is further evidence of cayenne's competence in treating hypertension: "Several years ago I was on Aldomet for high blood pressure, despite taking a variety of food supplements. I went to a health lecture on folk cures and heard about cayenne (hot red pepper) as a possible aid in controlling blood pressure problems. It worked wonders for me. For the first time in years my pressure became normal. It had been as high as 240/120 and was usually 190/110, even with the medicine. I was able to stop the medication I had been on for years." — *F.C., Florida.*

Cayenne capsules can be purchased from your local health food store (take one to three daily). But for hypertension, a great way to take cayenne is to take two tablespoonfuls of red pepper and the same quantity of Celtic sea salt, beat them into a paste, and add half a pint of very sharp vinegar. The recommended dose for an adult is a tablespoonful every hour. This mixture is extremely acrimonious, but it does work wonders. If you can't handle the taste, stick with the capsules.

Other Foods and Herbs That Work

In addition to garlic, celery, and cayenne pepper, there are several other foods and herbs that are effective treatments for high blood pressure. They include:

Fish Oil Helps Arterial Flexibility

"A study conducted by Irish researchers shows the loss of arterial flexibility that naturally occurs as people age — which can increase the risk of heart attacks and strokes — can be checked by the use of fish-oil supplements.

"In the study, 20 people were given 10 fish-oil supplements in capsule form or an olive-oil equivalent capsule for a six-week period. The olive-oil supplement was administered for six weeks, then the fish-oil supplement was given for the next six weeks.

"The results showed a marked improvement in the ability of the subject's arteries to stretch in response to blood pressure changes during the time the fish oil capsules were administered. From this case study, it seems this increased arterial flexibility is probably due to the fish-oil supplement's effect on the arteries." (*Let's Live*, 3/95; *Arteriosclerosis and Thrombosis*, 9/94)

Apple Cider Vinegar

The most effective way to treat high blood pressure with apple cider vinegar is to mix one or two teaspoons of it into a glass of water and *sip* with each meal. This remedy has been known to reduce blood pressure by 20 to 40 points within a half hour of eating a high-protein meal. If desired, an equal amount of raw honey may be added to the recipe.

Chervil

No clinical studies have been found to support claims that this herb cures hypertension, but many herbalists swear by it. Chervil is often used as an expectorant, a stimulant, and a digestive. But it is most persistently recognized for its ability to lower blood pressure. Those who use chervil for this purpose usually drink an infusion of the leaves and flowers.

Chives

Chives, like garlic, are another member of the onion family that helps lower blood pressure. They have the same sulfur-rich oil found in all the members of this family that is responsible for its flavor and medicinal properties. However, the amount of oil in chives is much less than that found in garlic or even in onions, so large quantities of the herb are required for the desired effect. This one is probably not strong enough to be used alone, but is ideal for use as a supplement to the other herbs.

Fish

Researcher Peter Singer, Ph.D., of Berlin, Germany said that his blood pressure dropped from 140/90 to 100/70 after he "started eating a small can of mackerel fillets every day." Dr. Singer found that the oil from fatty fish (i.e., salmon, mackerel, herring, sardines, and tuna) is as effective in reducing blood pressure as the commonly prescribed medication Inderal.

And when the two are taken together, they work better than either does by itself. That means if you're on blood pressure medication, adding a fish oil supplement to your diet may let you reduce the dosage of medication; and reduce the degree of its side effects. Fish oil also works similarly with propranolol or a thiazide diuretic.

Dr. Howard Knapp of Vanderbilt University confirmed these findings in a new study published in the *New England Journal of Medicine* (320,16:1037). Knapp's research "found that dietary supplementation with high doses of fish oil given for one month lowered blood pressure in men with mild essential hypertension, whereas a lower dose of fish oil, the same amount of safflower oil, or a mixture of saturated and unsaturated oils produced no significant change."

University of Cincinnati researchers studied the effects of fish oil on high blood pressure and determined that taking 2,000 milligrams of omega-3 fatty acids every day for three months was enough to substantially lower blood pressure levels. In some cases, the reduction was enough to eliminate the need for medication.

Jean Carper gives further evidence of fish oil's ability to reduce blood pressure in her book *Food: Your Miracle Medicine.* She cites a Danish study that suggests "a minimum of three servings of fish a week to control blood pressure. Investigators found that adding fish oil to the diet of those who ate fish three or more times a week *did not reduce blood pressure further.* However, doses of fish oil did depress blood pressure in those who did not eat that much fish. Thus it appears that fish eaten three times a week supplies enough omega-3 oil to control blood pressure in most people, which suggests high blood pressure is partly due to a 'fish deficiency.' Other components of seafood, such as potassium and selenium, may also contribute to lowering blood pressure."

Hawthorn

In Europe and Asia, many physicians use hawthorn extracts to help reduce high blood pressure. And its use has been affirmed in many scientific studies. Dr. Michael T. Murray, author of *Natural Alternatives to Over-the-Counter and Prescription Drugs*, says, "Hawthorn's action in lowering blood pressure is quite unique, in that it does so through a combination of many diverse actions. Specifically, it dilates the larger blood vessels, inhibits ACE similarly to the drug captopril, and increases the functional capacity of the heart....

"The dosage of hawthorn depends on the type of preparation and source material. Standardized extracts available in American health food stores are the preferred form for medicinal purposes. The dosage for a hawthorn extract (standardized to contain 1.8 percent vitexin-4'-rhamnoside or 10 percent procyanidins) would be 100 to 250 milligrams three times daily. Unlike synthetic drugs, hawthorn extracts are without side effects and are extremely well tolerated.

"The blood pressure-lowering effects of hawthorn extracts generally require up to two weeks before manifesting themselves. It appears this time is necessary to achieve adequate tissue concentrations of the flavonoids."

Lelord Kordel says that the Russian heart patients in the Caucasus Mountains use the hawthorn berry to make a fresh heart tonic every day. The directions are simple: "Pour two cups of boiling water over three tablespoonfuls of hawthorn berries. Cover and let stand overnight until midday in a very warm place (over a pilot light is fine). Strain the infusion through a fine mesh sieve or cloth, squeezing all juice from the berries.

"Dose: One cup, taken with meals at least twice a day. For a three-cup-a-day treatment, increase the formula accordingly.

"When fresh hawthorn berries are not available, the dried or powdered fruit can be obtained in many herb and health-food shops."

Another way to take hawthorn is to drink two cups of hawthorn tea daily made with the leaves and flowers and a small amount of valerian roots.

Olive Oil

Olive oil is becoming increasingly popular as a natural treatment for heart problems. In *Food: Your Miracle Medicine*, Jean Carper gives ample proof that olive oil is a must for hypertensives: "A study by researchers at Stanford Medical School of 76 middle-aged men with high blood pressure a few years ago concluded that the amount of monounsaturated fat in three tablespoons of olive oil a day could lower systolic pressure about nine points and diastolic pressure about six points. More remarkable, a University of Kentucky study found that a mere two-thirds of a tablespoon of olive oil daily reduced blood pressure by about five systolic points and four diastolic points in men. In a recent Dutch study, eating high amounts of olive oil drove down blood pressure slightly, even in those with normal pressure.

"Further, a major analysis of the diets of nearly 5,000 Italians noted that those eating the most olive oil had lower blood pressure by three or four points, especially men...."

Onion

The onion contains many of the same medicinal values as garlic, but with smaller doses of the antibacterial and antifungal components. Many scientific experiments have found that raw onions will have a lowering effect on mildly high blood pressure. One experiment, in fact, found that rats injected with an onion extract had significantly lower blood pressure than those in the control group.

Other research has recently confirmed a long held belief of naturalists that onions help clear the arteries of fatty deposits by increasing the production of high-density lipoproteins. As we mentioned at the beginning of this report, these deposits are partially responsible for an elevated blood pressure.

Rice

High blood pressure that is due to the diminishing elasticity of the blood vessels and not kidney disease or some other ailment can be easily corrected by a rice diet. Dr. H.C.A. Vogel explains in his book *The Nature Doctor* that "rice is a medicinal food, which provides surprisingly good results, but you must be sure to use brown unpolished rice, for this is more beneficial and valuable than the more common refined white rice. If you cannot obtain brown rice, although this is unlikely, two commercially prepared rice packages, 'Uncle Ben's' and

'Avorio' may serve as a compromise, because both of these brands still retain many of the important minerals found in brown rice....

"It is a proven fact that a diet of wholegrain rice promotes normal blood pressure. As it regulates low as well as high pressure, it would be wrong not to give it a chance for either of these problems. Not long ago I received a letter from a friend in Germany to whom I had recommended a wholegrain rice diet for his very high blood pressure. He had followed my advice and was able to report excellent results.

"He remained on the recommended diet for 10 weeks and found that he had lost weight and that his blood pressure had gone down from 230 to 190. This result alone was most encouraging. He then took a two-week vacation, at the end of which his pressure had fallen even further, this time to 170. Let me add that this patient is already 63 years old and it is especially interesting to note that he obtained such splendid results without the aid of any medication — simply by following a diet of wholegrain rice, cottage cheese, and salads...."

Serpentwood

Botanist James Duke, Ph.D., states in the *CRC Handbook of Medicinal Herbs* that serpentwood's "great value lies in its not requiring to be administered in critical dosages, rare side effects, non-habit-forming, without withdrawal symptoms, or contraindication."

Serpentwood has a 4,000 year history of use in India and has been used to treat insomnia, hyperglycemia, hypochondria, and certain mental disorders. But it is primarily used in treating hypertension.

Dr. William A.R. Thomson wrote in *Herbs That Heal*, "It had become incorporated into the folklore of India to such an extent that it was regularly chewed by the holy men of the country seeking tranquillity for their meditations, and Gandhi is said to have been a regular drinker of a tea made from it."

But according to the *Illustrated Encyclopedia of Herbs*, Western society wasn't interested in the herb, "even when its active principles were isolated by Indian chemists, or when it was prescribed to lower blood pressure by Indian physicians. But in 1949, an Indian cardiologist, Dr. R.J. Vakil, wrote an article about serpentwood in the *British Heart Journal*. Within a few years, scouts for the pharmaceutical industry were scouring the tropics for *Rauvolfia serpentina* and its relatives."

More Help for High Blood Pressure

We've discussed a wide variety of natural remedies to help you deal with high blood pressure. But there are other treatments that may help. In fact, there is one particular vitamin that is an effective preventive, as well as remedy, for high blood pressure.

It is niacin, one of the components of the vitamin B-complex. Niacin is found in wheat germ, brains, liver, lentils, avocados, and many other foods.

According to Lelord Kordel, author of *Health the Easy Way*, "Niacin is particularly effective in preventing and relieving a certain type of high blood pressure which is very common — that linked to nerves and nervousness. We have seen that the blood vessels, as well as the heart, are equipped with nerves. When these nerves are insulted or undernourished they may cause the blood vessels to become taut, thus raising the blood pressure above normal. As a specific remedy for high blood pressure of this type, I recommend abundant quantities of niacin in the daily diet. If the food sources of niacin mentioned above do not appeal to you, or are not easily available, niacin in concentrated form will be found both convenient and economical."

When taken in a sufficient dose (100-200 mg), niacin produces a dramatic reaction. According to Dr. Andrew Weil, author of *Natural Health, Natural Medicine,* "About 10 minutes after you swallow it, a sensation of prickly heat begins on the top of the head. This quickly develops into a wave of heat and redness that spreads down the whole body from the head to the feet.... After another 10 minutes the skin becomes blotchy instead of solid red, and the sensation becomes more itchy and crawly. All effects disappear 30 to 45 minutes after taking the vitamin. Some people find this reaction interesting and pleasant; others can't stand it.

"The niacin flush is the result of dilation of blood vessels in the skin due to the vitamin's effect on arteries and the nerves that regulate them." The reaction is harmless and generally has a positive effect on high blood pressure.

Dr. Weil adds this warning: "You will often see niacinamide, a closely related substance, on shelves next to niacin. Niacinamide has the same vitamin activity, but does not cause flushing. However, it is ineffective for the treatment of circulatory problems or elevated cholesterol. Do not use it."

Conclusion

As you can see, there are several natural remedies that have a long history of success for treating high blood pressure. These are not quack cures that don't work, but are legitimate treatments for a deadly disease you can administer at home.

Best of all, they can be taken with the drugs you are already on, or with each other, without any adverse effects. But if they don't work, you're no worse off — something that can't be said for most of the drugs your doctor will prescribe for you. And the difference they make in your cooking will make dinnertime a much more enjoyable part of your day.

A healthy circulatory system is a major key to living a long healthy life. And the better we take care of our blood, the better our health will be. A simple one-two step won't fix problems that have taken years to develop.

(Editor's note: High blood pressure can also be reduced by a doctor-administered treatment called EDTA chelation therapy. This alternative therapy is extremely effective for most heart-related problems. You can read about it in The Chelation Answer *by Dr. Morton Walker. It's available for $16.90 from Second Opinion Publishing. Call 800-728-2288. For the name of a doctor in your area who administers this therapy, call the American College for the Advancement of Medicine (ACAM) at 800-532-3688 or the International Oxidative Medicine Association (IOMA) at 405-478-4266.)*

Chapter 13

Questions and Answers

Poor Circulation

Q. My doctor says that the numbness and tingling sensations I feel in my legs are due to poor circulation. If this is true, what can I do about it?

A. The adult human heart weighs approximately a half pound and pumps over five hundred gallons of blood a day through an intricate system of arteries, veins, and capillaries. If, for some reason, the blood flow to a particular part of the body (usually the extremities) is not adequate, that area becomes weakened. Symptoms of poor circulation range anywhere from a minor tingling sensation, to numbness, to (in extreme situations) gangrene.

Problems with minor circulatory problems (as with most health problems) often stem from a poor diet. Dr. Bernard Jensen, author of *Foods That Heal*, says that every bodily "disorder responds well to appropriate vegetable juices." Dr. Jensen asserts that blackberry juice is one of the finest builders of the blood, but that it can cause constipation. To minimize the constipation effect, he recommends mixing the blackberry juice with beet juice. Another juice that works well for poor circulation is a mixture of parsley and alfalfa juice with pineapple juice. The parsley acts as a strong blood builder and purifier.

The final juice Dr. Jensen recommends is grape juice with one egg yolk added to it. Whey and soy milk can also be added to this mixture to make "a wonderful tonic for the blood."

Heart Cramps

Q. My husband suffers from angina. The doctor wants to put him on some strong antibiotics, but I know that strong side effects usually accompany strong medications. Is there anything I can do to help him when the pain hits?

A. Modern medicine generally treats heart cramps in cases of angina pectoris with radical medicines like amyl nitrite or Trinitrin (nitroglycerin). "There is, however, an old and exceedingly simple remedy which is quite easy to come by," says Dr. H.C.A. Vogel in his book, *The Nature Doctor*. This longtime country remedy has been in use for centuries, but has been all but forgotten today. It "relieves the spasms without any side effects or complications. The same remedy is also good for asthma attacks."

Here's what you do: "Take some fermented cider, the older the better, heat it until it reaches the boiling point and quickly remove it from the heat. Then soak some towels in the hot liquid and place them, as hot as the patient can bear, on both arms, covering each arm completely. The heat plus the fruit acids of the hot cider will decongest the heart circulation, soothe the blood vessels and the nervous system, and relieve the cramps. The effect of this simple, natural treatment can be reinforced by placing a hot linseed, hay flower, or lemon balm compress over the heart at the same time. Linseed is the best choice for this purpose."

Raynaud's disease

Q. I have Raynaud's disease, a circulatory disorder which so far just affects my fingers. After I have an attack and when the blood flow returns to my fingers, it is very painful. Sometimes I am left with a tender 'bruise'-like area for days. My doctor just advises me to 'wear gloves.' Are there any vitamins or minerals I could be taking that would help this?"

A. As you said, Raynaud's disease is an uncomfortable and sometimes disabling circulatory disorder that is characterized by the constriction and spasm of the smaller vascular system. The symptoms are usually noticed in the fingers, but occasionally occur in the nose, tongue, and feet. Your tender bruise area is probably a response to the cold or an emotionally stressful situation.

As far as treating the disease with vitamins and minerals, the most successful supplement has been vitamin E. Gradually building up your dosage to 900 to 1,500 I.U. daily has totally alleviated the symptoms of this disease in many cases. You might also take a magnesium supplement (200 mg. three times daily).

Scientists recently revealed an at-home treatment that helps relieve the symptoms of Raynaud's. According to the *Book of Proven Home Remedies and Natural Healing Secrets*, the steps are as follows:

"1. Fill two bowls with water of about 120 degrees. Place one bowl in a cold area (either a room or outdoors) and place the other in a warm room.

"2. Dress lightly, as you would for room temperature. In the warm room, put both hands in the 120-degree water for two to five minutes.

"3. Wrap the hands in a towel and go to the cold room. Again put both hands in the 120-degree water for two to five minutes.

"4. Repeat step 2 — put hands in warm water in the warm room for two to five minutes.

"5. Repeat this procedure three to six times a day for a total of about 50 trials."

But the simplest form of treatment that has seen tremendous results is to swing your arms around in giant circles. You'll look like you're trying to do a windmill imitation, but it has worked for some people in as few as 90 seconds.

Heart Attacks

Q. My husband has had two heart attacks. Every now and then he has shortness of breath that scares me terribly. He is currently taking vitamins C, E, and A, as well as several mineral supplements. Are there any supplements he's missing?

A. Yes, there's one very important one missing from his regimen. It's coenzyme Q10 or CoQ10. It's available from most health food stores and is a must for heart disease patients. Dr. Julian Whitaker relates the following story to show how important this supplement can be:

"Maria Irene Silva was 49 years old when she had three heart attacks, one after another, and was diagnosed with early stage cardiomyopathy, a progressive weakening of the heart. At that time her ejection fraction, the percent of blood the heart chambers pump out with each beat, was almost normal at 48 percent.

"She did fairly well until March of 1994, when she began gasping for air.... She was in congestive heart failure. Her ejection fraction had dropped all the way down to 21 percent and she was diagnosed with advanced dilated idiopathic cardiomyopathy. Six months later her ejection fraction had fallen to the dangerously low level of 14 percent. She was told that her condition was irreversible, incurable, and that her only hope for improvement was a heart transplant, which would cost about $300,000.

"At about that time, ... Maria's husband read about coenzyme Q10, and started giving her 900 mg a day, along with other natural supplements. To everyone's surprise, her ejection fraction rose to 39 percent, and the two of them believe that 'God has made a miracle due to the CoQ10.'

"Maria has continued taking coenzyme Q10, and continues to improve. She is fully functional, able to do housework, and walks for 30 minutes a day. She has lost 43 pounds of water, and says she feels better than she has in years. Regardless of what her next heart evaluation shows, she is certainly no candidate for a heart transplant." (*Health & Healing*; 2/95)

Section 4

Cancer

Chapter 14

Can You Effectively Prevent and Treat Cancer at Home?

In 1992, I lost my mom to ovarian cancer. Her tumor was discovered in the spring of 1991, and in the ensuing months she followed the established line for medical treatment of ovarian cancer: surgery, chemotherapy, radiation. Unfortunately, ovarian cancer is a very hard cancer that is resistant to every known form of conventional medicine.

Needless to say, winning the war against cancer is something I take very seriously. And writing an article about preventing and treating cancer is not something I can enter into lightly or flippantly. I know what's on the line for those suffering from the disease. And I also know the disease has affected just about everyone who will read this article in some way.

I recognize that some forms of cancer can be destroyed with a high degree of success by conventional medicine. This article is by no means intended to discredit these treatments or discourage you from using them.

However, conventional medicine will be the first to admit that we are losing this war against most cancers. That's reason enough to stress prevention. But is the situation hopeless when you or a loved one is stricken with cancer and you know the conventional therapies won't work? In many cases, I don't believe it is.

More Research on Cancer Protection From Fruits and Vegetables

We've seen how fruits and vegetables fight against cancer development. Now we have even more evidence: "Researchers at the Athens Medical School (Greece) and the Harvard School of Public Health have just completed a major study aimed at determining the effect of diet on the risk of developing breast cancer. Their investigation involved 820 women with breast cancer and 1,548 controls. The researchers found that women who ate large quantities of fruits had a 35 percent lower risk of developing breast cancer than did women who consumed only small amounts. The risk factor among women who ate lots of vegetables was 46 percent lower than among women who only ate few vegetables.... A high margarine consumption was found to significantly increase the risk of developing breast cancer. There was no indication that the consumption of butter is related to the risk of breast cancer." (*International Health News*, March 1995; *Journal of the National Cancer Institute*, January 18, 1995.)

Can We Find All the Causes?

Cancer can almost always be linked to environmental causes; either what is around us or what we eat, usually the latter. Pollution, electrical fields, pesticides, preservatives (and other pollutants in our diet), and many other manmade and natural toxins have been found to be carcinogenic. We've really just scratched the surface, though, in finding all the causes of cancer.

Research is important, but I don't think we'll ever find all the things that cause this dreadful disease. Because of this, it's crucial to fight the war against cancer with a strong defense — a defense that can withstand the constant bombardment of unknown toxins.

More Cancer Protection

A new study indicates that black tea is a potent protector against certain types of cancer. The study was conducted by Dr. Chung Yang of Rutgers University and showed that the popular tea helps protect against skin, lung, and esophagus cancer.

According to Dr. Robert Atkins's analysis, "When mice were exposed to carcinogenic ultraviolet radiation, those that had been given green or black tea to drink had 70 percent fewer tumors than the mice given only water to drink. Dr. Yang says he believes a class of chemicals called catechins is responsible for the cancer-fighting ability of the drink." (*Health Revelations*, 2/95)

The Best Offense Is a Good Defense

Fortunately, when God created us, He gave us a strong defense mechanism in the immune system. But the immune system can be beaten down and defeated if it's

---

Relief from Pain of Mouth Cancer

"Professor Linda Bartoshuk's research into anesthetizing the tongue with the fiery compound from chilies (capsaicin) to block pain has led to a dramatic pain-relief treatment for cancer patients.

"It utilizes a mixture of Betty Crocker taffy and cayenne pepper, according to a report in the current (January/February 1995) issue of *The Sciences*.

"Bartoshuk and Yale colleague Ann Berger, of the oncology department, served the 'hot taffy ... to nine cancer patients with mouth lesions,' reports *The Sciences*. 'On a pain scale from one to 10 — 10 being the worst ever experienced — a single dose of the candy reduced the patients' average pain from six to 1.5 for several hours. No other oral irritant exhibits capsaicin's pain-deadening power, a fact that Bartoshuk is currently reconfirming with a placebo study using black pepper.'

"'It is an incredible effect for a trivial intervention. It's easy on the patient, and it's cheap,' Bartoshuk says. 'What we have done with this approach to (oral) pain is simply more effective than anything that anyone else has done for these patients.'" (*Cancer Biotechnology Weekly*, 1/9/95)

not given the proper support. That's where your part comes in.

The role of diet in the prevention and treatment of cancer is absolutely vital. There are numerous studies proving this, including one study that demonstrated how the rate of breast cancer for Japanese women is almost nonexistent until they migrate to the U.S. and begin

---

Broccoli and Cancer

Scientists have found a chemical in broccoli that seems to inhibit the growth of cancer cells. According to a report in the *Atlanta Journal*, "The newly isolated substance stimulates production of enzymes that can break down carcinogens, including the female hormone estrogen, Texas A&M University researchers reported in today's issue of the *Journal of the National Cancer Institute.*... Some experts think estrogen exposure may play a role in some breast cancers....

"Instead of suggesting that eating sufficient amounts of broccoli will ward off breast cancer, the experiment illustrates the vigorous druglike properties that may be found in the natural products contained in plant cells, other researchers said."

Don't listen to the "other researchers." Eat plenty of broccoli as part of a good diet. Eat even more broccoli if you have a family history of breast cancer. It sure couldn't hurt. (*Atlanta Journal*, 12/7/94)

eating a typical American diet. Then their rate of breast cancer increases dramatically.

What follows are several simple recommendations that will help you strengthen your immune system for the prevention and treatment of cancer. All of them can be done at home and most can be done in conjunction with other treatments.

What Should You Be Eating?

Grapes: Back in 1928, Johanna Brandt wrote a book called *The Grape Cure.* She writes: "Cancer is the death and disintegration of a given part in a living body. I am convinced this is due to the presence of corrosive substances with which nature is unable to cope.

"Fasting does not effectually eliminate them. If the cancer is not too far advanced, a diet of raw fruits and vegetables may save the patient, but in extreme cases something is required by which those corroding, irritating

---

Black Pepper Helps Prevent Cancer

"Researchers have found that common black pepper can protect against chemically induced cancer.

"Animal studies have shown that when up to two percent of the diet consisted of black pepper, it facilitated a detoxification process within the liver. Chemical analysis also showed it lowered the oxidation of fats." (*Cancer Letter*, 93;72:5-9; *Alternatives*, December 1994)

---

substances may be quickly dissolved and expelled — something by which at the same time the strength of the patient may be nourished.

Grapes are loaded with ellagic acid and other healthful chemicals that allow this fruit to effectually answer all three of these requirements. Researchers have found that a diet of Concord grapes was effective in slowing tumor growth in mice — a fact Johanna Brandt was aware of over 65 years ago.

If you have cancer, Brandt says a grape diet can cure it in many instances by following the proper procedure:

1. Fast for two or three days and drink nothing but cold water.

2. On the first morning after the fast, drink one or two glasses of cold water first thing.

3. Half an hour later begin chewing on the grapes (and seeds) "and swallow only a *few* of them as food and roughage.

4. "Starting at 8:00 a.m. and having a grape meal every two hours till 8:00 p.m., this would give seven meals daily. This is kept up for a week or two, even a month or two in chronic cases of long-standing." Not longer under any circumstances." (Any variety of grapes will do — purple, green, red, white, or blue.)

5. Begin with small quantities and work your way up to a minimum of one pound daily and a maximum of four pounds. (If you eat more than four pounds, allow three hours between meals. However, small quantities are the most effective.)

6. If you loathe the grapes, fast for another day and resume the diet.

According to Brandt, this system will cause you to lose strength "due to the presence of poisons in the

Licorice Root Prevents Breast Cancer and Other Ailments

"According to *Health Line*, researchers from around the globe at a recent Designer Foods Symposium, extolled the many benefits of licorice root extract. One reason for the growing interest in this sweet substance is the potential number of beneficial compounds it may contain.... Following are some of the promising effects of using licorice root extract:

"* It is intensely sweet-tasting, yet it contains no calories. Thus, it may hold promise for flavoring 'sweet-tooth satisfying' foods that do not contain high amounts of sugar.

"* While non-toxic itself, licorice root extract has shown promising activity against HIV (human immunodeficiency virus) in clinical human trials in Japan.

"* Licorice phytochemicals have been shown to be effective in preventing breast cancer when used in animal model experiments.

"* It is thought to be one of the best anti-inflammatories and is currently available for use in ulcer treatment in Europe.

"* It may have properties that prevent tooth decay and gum disease. These are two major 'plagues' that cause pain, cost money, and may undercut proper nutrition." (*Let's Live*, 3/95)

system. The patient continues to weaken under the grape diet and under the complete fast, until the poison has been expelled. Then, without a change of diet, the patient returns to strength and in some cases even puts on weight."

Once your strength returns, slowly begin to add fresh fruits, tomatoes, and sour milk or cottage cheese to your diet. Add only one fruit per day for a few days, eating one type per meal. Then add the other foods gradually. After a few days of this, add any other foods that can be eaten raw: vegetables, nuts, butter, honey, olive oil, salads, etc.

Onions, Garlic, and Chili Peppers: Many of you probably try to avoid these herbs because of their penchant for causing bad breath. But don't let a little halitosis discourage the use of these fantastic cancer fighters.

A study performed in the Shandong Province in China (where stomach cancer rates were high) found that patients who ate at least three ounces of onions and garlic a day were 40 percent as likely to develop stomach cancer as those who ate only one ounce. They also found that the more onions and garlic the patients ate, the better the protective effect.

Nearly 40 years ago, researchers discovered that garlic had the incredible ability to delay the development of malignant tumors and in many cases completely prevent their formation. Both onions and garlic contain sulfurous compounds that block the growth of cancer in laboratory tests.

According to the National Cancer Institute, "In the county of Georgia where Vidalia onions are grown, the

Obesity and Cancer of the Esophagus

"The incidence of adenocarcinoma of the esophagus among white men has tripled between 1976 and 1990. Researchers at the National Cancer Institute have now found that obese men are three times more likely to develop esophageal cancer than are men with a normal body weight. The researchers also discovered that a high intake of fruits and vegetables, particularly cruciferous vegetables, is protective against esophageal cancer. Fiber (from fruit and vegetables) was also found to be highly protective with a higher consumption yielding increased protection. Cigarette smoking, alcohol consumption, a history of ulcers and a low annual income were found to be significant additional risk factors for the development of adenocarcinoma of the esophagus." (*International Health News*, March 1995)

stomach cancer rate is only half that of other Georgia counties, and one-third that of the rest of the United States."

"Similarly," says Jean Carper, author of *Food: Your Miracle Medicine*, "John Milner, head of nutrition at Penn State University, blocked 70 percent of breast tumors in mice by feeding them fresh garlic. In humans, studies show that those who eat more onions and garlic are less prone to various cancers."

Nutty Cancer Fighter

"Researchers at Roswell Park Cancer Institute recently observed that animals fed Brazil nuts ... showed an increased cancer resistance. The tropical nut contains exceptionally high levels of selenium, a trace element with potent anticancer properties.

"Animals fed a diet enriched with Brazil nuts were better able to resist tumors than those fed a walnut-enriched diet (walnuts are low in selenium). The researchers then compared the Brazil nut's anticancer potential to selenium supplements and found the nut to be 'just as powerful as sodium selenite, if not more so, at similar levels of dietary selenium intake.'

"Modern diets often lack selenium because agricultural soils are widely deficient in it. Tuna, chicken, pork, and beef contain some selenium, but typically 100 to 300 times less per gram than Brazil nuts. Garlic grown in selenium-enriched soil is a good source, though still not as rich as Brazil nuts. (Buying organic may be your best bet for getting adequate levels of selenium in your vegetables and herbs. You can also grow your own — certain agricultural agencies can help you figure out if your soil needs a selenium 'amendment.')

"Eating a few Brazil nuts a day in the context of a balanced diet will bolster selenium reserves. Vitamin E, which is amply supplied by seeds, nuts, and whole grains, works in tandem with selenium to promote the body's resistance to disease. The Roswell Park researchers warn against going overboard with Brazil nuts, however, since selenium is toxic at high levels — a small handful a day is plenty." (*Natural Health*, 3-4/95)

Chili peppers were once thought to cause stomach cancer, but according to *Health* magazine, "people in Mexico are relatively unlikely to develop stomach cancer, although they eat lots of chilies." Peppers also prevent cigarette smoke from grabbing onto DNA, which can cause lung and other cancers.

Tea: Tea (green or black) contains polyphenols, which is a much stronger antioxidant than either Vitamin E or Vitamin C. Drinking several cups of green tea each day may be one way to provide our cells with antioxidants to prevent cancer. When cells turn cancerous, polyphenols seem to prevent them from multiplying and

---

Does Olive Oil Help Breast Cancer?

According to a new study reported in the *Journal of the National Cancer Institute*, it does. The study "evaluated 820 women with breast cancer and 1,548 control women to compare the relationship of using olive oil, margarine, and other foods with breast cancer. The results showed that women who eat vegetables had a reduction of 12 percent in the incidence of breast cancer; women who consumed fruits showed a reduction of eight percent; and, other food groups that were consumed showed no significant change in the incidence of breast cancer. However, women who consumed olive oil showed the most significant reduction." (*Let's Live*, June 1995)

also help eliminate carcinogens from the body. Studies have repeatedly shown a reduction in the number and size of cancerous tumors in laboratory animals suggesting that tea may be protective against many types of cancer. This evidence is supported by studies of people in the Shizuoka Prefecture in Japan, who have less stomach cancer than people who live in other parts of the country. Their major dietary difference is a greater consumption of tea. The extract of green tea has even been used topically to reduce skin cancer.

The latest tea to hit the market as a cancer treatment is Essiac tea. Thousands of people claim to have been healed by the tea, but modern medicine still shuns it. One patient had lip cancer and was given radium treatments. His lip became so swollen he could see it over the end of his nose. The pain was excruciating and he soon had to leave his job. After one injection of Essiac, Tony felt immediate relief and was back on the job after drinking the tea for six months.

Essiac is easy to take and should be taken by cancer patients at any stage. Drink two fluid ounces three times a day for at least 12 consecutive weeks, without interruption. You've got to give it time to work.

Essiac tea is available at your local health food store or from Essiac International at 800-668-4559. Aloe Vera Products from North America also sells the tea (800-998-2563). It's fairly expensive, but well worth the price. From Essiac International you'll pay $39.50 for one ounce of dried tea, which will make about one to two quarts of tea. Aloe Vera Products from North America sells two ounces for $19.95 (makes four quarts) and New Action Products (716-873-3738) sells a tea-making kit for $35 (makes eight quarts).

If you would like more information about Essiac, I suggest you read *The Essiac Report* by Richard Thomas (available from The Alternative Treatment Information Network, 1244 Ozeta Terrace, Los Angeles, CA 90069, 800-446-3063, for $19.95 plus $1.25 S&H).

Other Foods: There are many other foods that are effective cancer fighters. Eating a diet that includes large amounts of cabbage, soybeans, carrots, tomatoes, fish, broccoli, collard greens, and fruits (especially oranges and lemons) will greatly reduce your cancer risks. If you already have cancer, these foods will help your body eradicate the disease.

For prevention, "nobody really knows the best anticancer dose of fruits and vegetables, but at least two fruits and three vegetables a day of various kinds are a goal to aim for. Adding more fruits and vegetables to a typical diet is likely to cut your chances of cancer," concludes Jean Carper.

Chapter 15

Help for Specific Cancers

The role of diet in preventing and treating cancer is absolutely vital. We just saw how important it is for us to include certain foods in our diet as preventive measures, and how other foods can be used to actively destroy cancer tumors.

Nutrition experts disagree on why foods have this effect on tumors. Some say that cancer is the result of poisons in the body accumulating around the weakest organs. Others, like Elizabeth Holihan, N.D., author of *Human Fuel*, say, "Cancer is the crystallization of resources, stored within cells. The body is storing crystallized resources in cells because it needs them, but can't make use of them, without other resources that are inadequately provided."

Either way, cancer is usually caused by a deficiency of nutrients the body needs to operate properly. However, there are some cancers that are more affected by diet than others. Cervical cancer is almost always caused by sexually transmitted diseases and lung cancer is typically the result of smoking. But, in general, you can call cancer a disease of bad habits.

Walking Off Breast Cancer

"A study of more than 1,000 women age 40 and younger has found that moderate, regular physical activity may also cut the odds of developing premenopausal breast cancer.

"Researchers at the University of Southern California (USC) School of Medicine in Los Angeles found that:

"Women who exercised about four hours a week reduced their risk of developing breast cancer at an early age by as much as 58 percent.

"Those who worked out just one to three hours a week lowered their risk by 20 percent to 30 percent. The women were involved in activities such as swimming, jogging, racket sports, aerobic dance, and brisk walking.

"Women who exercised during the 10 years after their first period seemed to reap the greatest benefit. But even late-comers to physical activity experienced a payoff. 'We still saw a very strong protective effect among women who became active in their late 20s and 30s,' says lead study author Leslie Bernstein, Ph.D., professor of preventive medicine at USC.

"Women with a 'spotty' workout record — those who exercise vigilantly for two or three years, then slacked off for several years, only to resume exercising later on — also achieved a significant amount of protection." (*Parents*, 3/95)

Of the cancers caused largely by bad dietary habits, breast, colon, and prostate cancers are the most common.

Obviously, prevention is the best way to deal with these cancers, but what should you do if the doctor gives you the dreaded news that you have cancer? The difference between prevention and treatment is very small. What will prevent the tumor from growing in the first place will usually destroy the cancer once it is in place.

What follows is not an exhaustive list of things to do, but hopefully it will point you in the right direction. Also know that while chemotherapy, radiation, and surgery may not be the best way to go, this is not intended to replace any treatment given by your doctor. Rather, these steps should be done in conjunction with any supervised treatment you may decide to receive.

Breast Cancer

The statistics say one of every nine women will suffer breast cancer, but the fear of the disease hits every one of those nine women. Here are some tips from *Women's Health Letter* (July 1995) that might help in your fight against breast cancer:

Please Pass on the Sugar

"Several studies have linked high sugar consumption to increased breast cancer risk. This is not surprising when you consider the massive amounts of glucose cancer cells need to thrive — 10 times more than normal cells.

"An epidemiologic survey reported in the *Journal of Medical Hypothesis* reviewed breast cancer rates for 21

Nutrients Fight Precancerous Lesions

"Leukoplakia is a relatively common condition of the oral cavity. The whitish plaques that give rise to the name "leukoplakia" can become malignant and are therefore considered precancerous.

"Because selenium is known to have anti-cancer effects, this trace mineral was given to 18 patients with leukoplakia or other precancerous lesions of the mouth. Each patient received 300 mcg/day of selenium for 12 weeks. In two cases (11.1 percent), the lesions disappeared completely and in another five individuals, the leukoplakia shrank by more than 50 percent. Overall, 72 percent of the patients improved while receiving selenium and none became worse. After selenium was discontinued, the condition became worse in seven of the 18 patients....

"Studies published more than 40 years ago showed that vitamin A supplements also improve this condition and more recent research suggests that beta-carotene may be beneficial. Interestingly, each of these three nutrients has been found repeatedly to have anticancer effects.

"Experience has shown that, for many medical problems, a combination of nutrients is more effective than any single nutrient alone. Thus, it is likely that using selenium, vitamin A, and beta-carotene together would produce the best results for individuals with leukoplakia." (*Cancer Detection and Prevention*, 1991;15:491-494; *Nutrition & Healing*, April 1995)

countries. Based on their findings, the researchers concluded that high sucrose (sugar) intake is a major risk factor for the development of breast cancer in women over 45.

Antioxidants

"Women who want to lower their breast cancer risk should also boost the antioxidant content of their meals at every opportunity. Fruits and vegetables are a main source of antioxidants.

"In two Swedish studies reported in the *Archives of Internal Medicine*, researchers found a breast cancer decrease with a high intake of the antioxidant beta-carotene, the form of vitamin A found in many red, yellow, and orange fruits and vegetables. Green vegetables were also protective.... [If the cancer has developed, you may need to take large doses of specific supplements. Because each person has different needs, we recommend you do this under the supervision of a nutritionally trained doctor.]

Eat Plenty of Fiber

"If you experience constipation, upping your fiber intake should take care of the problem and will lower your breast cancer risk as well. Women with two or less bowel movements per week have 4.5 times the risk of precancerous breast changes than women whose frequency is greater than once per day, according to researchers from the University of California at San Francisco."

Reduce Your Risk of
Skin Cancer by 70 Percent

"Every year more than 500,000 white Americans are diagnosed with new cases of skin cancer. What can you do to protect yourself? In addition to following sun-safety guidelines, consider this: a Johns Hopkins University study showed that people who use any vitamins had less skin cancer than the control patients without skin cancer.

"The risk for skin cancer was reduced by 70 percent for those people who regularly took supplements, particularly multivitamins and antioxidants. The more regularly people took these supplements, and the higher the doses, the more protection.

"Be aware that high amounts of vitamin A should not be taken by children or pregnant women. However, beta-carotene, which is found in produce and turns into vitamin A in your body, is very safe in larger amounts. If you are pregnant or trying to conceive, limit vitamin A to 5,000 IU a day.

"And remember that the safest form of all vitamins is found in good quality foods. Eat at least two healthy servings of vegetables a day — cooked or raw. If you sprinkle a few raw nuts or seeds in your breakfast cereal or on your salad, you'll be adding more natural vitamins. Perhaps a future study will include data from women who eat a diet high in antioxidants." (*Vitamin Nutrition Research Newsletter*, Roche Vitamins, Vol. 1, No. 2, December 1994; *Women's Health Letter*, July 1995)

Other foods you need to eat regularly include: cabbage, wheat bran, beans (pinto, garbanzo, black beans, and soybeans), and seafood.

In addition to diet changes, women who have breast cancer should take the following suggestions from *Herbal Healing for Women* by Rosemary Gladstar:

* Chaparral tincture: one teaspoon three times a day.
* Chaparral tablets: two tablets three times a day.
* Chlorophyll and/or wheat grass juice: one teaspoon three times a day.
* Blue-green algae: one teaspoon three times a day.
* Pau d'arco/echinacea tea: one cup three times a day.
* Reishi mushroom: three capsules three times a day.

There is now evidence that breast cancer may be linked to women wearing tight bras for extended periods of time. In their book *Dressed to Kill: The Link Between Breast Cancer and Bras* (Avery, 1995), Sydney Ross Singer and Soma Grismaijer discuss their findings on a revolutionary breast cancer theory. But Singer and Grismaijer are quick to recognize diet as the main defense against breast cancer.

Colon Cancer

Americans have dramatically increased their consumption of refined foods and sugar over the last 50 years and reduced their intake of fiber. As a result, we have seen a striking escalation in the colon cancer rates.

Researchers are finding that sugar alone reduces the transit time in the digestive tract and boosts the level of toxic substances in the tract.

According to *Alternatives* newsletter, "A group of patients on a diet containing 165 grams of sugar a day was compared to another group of patients eating only 60 grams a day. Not only did food move through the digestive tract slower in those on the high sugar diet, the total bile acids and stool concentrations of bile acids were greater (*Gut* 91;32:367-371)."

Finnish men consume nearly the same amount of fat as Americans, but have one-third the rate of colon cancer. Why? Researchers say the Finns eat large amounts of whole rye that provides protection from colon cancer. It's been well established that grains can greatly decrease the risk of colon cancer.

According to John Heinerman, author of *Heinerman's Encyclopedia of Fruits, Vegetables, and Herbs*, "The green juice from young barley shoots possesses strong anti-inflammatory activity.... And research conducted by Dr. Chiu-Nan Lai at the M.D. Anderson Hospital & Tumor Institute in Houston, Texas shows that extracts of wheat sprouts can modify, even decrease, the formation of cancer of the esophagus, stomach, liver, breast, and colon, if regularly used in the diet." You can purchase these cereal grasses in tablet form or bulk powder from Pines International, Inc. (P.O. Box 1107, Lawrence, KS 66044).

You also need to clean out your colon. The best way to do this is to take two Okra Pepsin tablets, called Nutri-Flax, three times a day. You can order these flax-meal supplements from Omega Nutrition in Canada (800-661-3529).

Other foods you need to eat include: cruciferous vegetables (cabbage, broccoli, cauliflower, brussels sprouts), fatty fish (mackerel, anchovies, salmon, and herring), apples, carrots, onions, peppers, soy, and yogurt.

If you suffer from ulcerative colitis, you may also want to supplement your diet with 400 mcg of folic acid. University of Chicago researchers found that people with ulcerative colitis who take folic acid supplements are half as likely to have precancerous cells in their colons.

Prostate Cancer

Prostate cancer is a very slow-growing cancer that usually hits elderly men, most of whom die of other causes without suffering any symptoms from the cancer. Because of this, many doctors will not recommend any treatment.

However, complete relief from prostate cancer and other problems of the prostate has been obtained by simply using natural herbs and vitamins. The following testimonial from *Natural Home Remedies* is just a taste of what researchers have found to be true:

"Two years ago, I was suffering from a severe prostate situation and I thought my days were numbered. The pain was incredible and I thought if this continued, I couldn't make it. My doctor gave me penicillin, but that didn't work. I went to three urologists, but that didn't help....

"Finally, after reading and doing research, I went on a self-healing campaign on my own.

"I cut out coffee, tea, diet soda, tomato juice, and tomatoes. I drank apple juice and cranberry juice. I took large doses of vitamin C, plus zinc and pumpkin seed capsules. I started exercising by playing golf, tennis, bike riding, and walking. I took hot baths twice a day.

"Today, a year later, I feel completely healed." — *J.D., Arizona.*

Perhaps one of the strongest cancer-fighting substances I've seen is beetroot. It not only works on prostate cancer, but on many different cancers, including breast and colon. Beetroot contains an ingredient that actively destroys tumors. According to John Heinerman, "One has to be careful with the amount of beets consumed at any given time. Certainly not because they're harmful, but rather due to their incredibly strong ability to quickly break up cancer in the body. A woman in her 30s who was treated with beetroot for breast cancer contracted a fever of 104 degrees F. due to the rapid breakdown of the tumors. In instances such as this, beets clean up the cancer faster than the liver is capable of processing all of the wastes dumped into it at any one time." Beetroot powder is available at most local health food stores.

Conclusion

You may have noticed that many of the specific recommendations for these cancers can also be used for the treatment of other cancers. That's not just a coincidence. Treating cancer takes a whole-body approach and most of these treatments help the body heal itself. But the list of natural healers doesn't stop here. There are many other natural methods you can safely use to prevent and treat cancer. Do a little research and you'll be amazed at what you can do at home.

Chapter 16
Old-Time Cures for Cancer

The cancer rate seems to be reaching epidemic proportions in many parts of the world, making the disease look like a relatively new scourge. But cancer has actually been around for thousands of years.

In the Old Testament, the Bible speaks of an Israelite king named Hezekiah who "became ill and was at the point of death." His affliction was simply called a boil, but because of the serious nature of the boil, many biblical scholars believe it was a tumor. The Lord told Isaiah to place "a poultice of figs" on the wound. He did as the Lord commanded and the king was healed and lived for another 15 years. (NIV, 2 Kings 20:1-7; Isaiah 38:21)

Now Japanese scientists have found that figs contain an active carcinostatic principle called benzaldehyde. According to *Natural Home Remedies* (Rodale, 1982), "Clinically, steam distillates of fig fruit reduced malignant human tumors by as much as 39 percent. Ironically, figs work better on human tumors than on mouse or rat tumors."

The *National Dispensatory* of 1880 revealed an interesting treatment for cancer. It was called red root, better known today as New Jersey tea. The settlers of the 13 colonies were introduced to this plant by the Indians and made infusions of green and dried leaves to make a beverage much like Chinese green tea. You already know about green tea's ability to treat cancer, but about red root the *Dispensatory* added: "The root is astringent, and

---

Lack of Sunlight Shown to Cause Ovarian Cancer

"It is known that the incidence of breast and colon cancer is higher in geographical areas which receive relatively little sunlight. Now researchers at the University of San Diego have found that American women aged 45 to 54 living in the northern U.S.A. are five times more likely to die from ovarian cancer than are women living in the southern states. The researchers believe that vitamin D protects against certain forms of cancer and speculate that the reason for the higher incidence of cancer at northern latitudes is a lack of vitamin D. Approximately 70 percent of an adult's vitamin D supply is generated by sunlight-induced photo-conversion of 7-dehydro-cholesterol to vitamin D_3 in the skin.... The use of sunscreens blocks the skin's absorption of UVB rays which are the rays needed for the photosynthesis of vitamin D." (*International Health News*, March 1995; *International Journal of Epidemiology*, December 1994)

was applied locally by the Cherokee Indians in gonorrhea and cancer."

Then in the early 20th century, Jethro Kloss found that diet and the application of heat can be very effective in treating cancer. But it wasn't until the 1970s that mainstream medicine grabbed onto the idea of treating cancer with temperatures above normal. A number of medical centers found that heat actually reduced cancerous tumors.

But Kloss also contributed to the treatment of cancer in the area of diet. He wrote in *Back to Eden* (Back to Eden Books, 1994):

"People used to think that meat was the great cause of cancer, but in my research I discovered that some people who ate no meat at all still developed cancer. I also found that people who did not eat meat, and with whose habits of diet I was well acquainted, also had cancer. They were eating refined food and bad combinations of food of such a nature that much waste matter accumulated in the system. This caused the different organs to become diseased and many times cancer resulted...."

Kloss' treatment of cancer is similar to the latter stages of Johanna Brandt's grape diet mentioned in chapter 14: "It is necessary to take a fruit diet of oranges, grapefruit, lemons, apples, cranberries, unsweetened blueberries, red raspberries, cherries, peaches, pears, ripe strawberries, avocados, pineapples, and tomatoes. All fruit should be well ripened on the tree or vine to be fully beneficial.

"Tomatoes should be eaten separately, not with other foods. Make a meal of them.... For the first 10 days ... it is advisable to take nothing but unsweetened fruit juices....

Do not mix the juice, but take different ones at different times.

"Never cook food in aluminum cooking utensils. Never eat fruit and vegetables at the same meal, nor drink fruit and vegetable juices at the same time.

"Get plenty of fresh air and exercise, outdoors in the sunshine if possible, to cleanse the lungs and increase the circulation...."

Modern medicine can do many wonderful things, but don't ignore the age-old wisdom of our ancestors. Even tough diseases like cancer can often be cured with their remedies.

Section 5

Digestive Problems

Chapter 17

40 Remedies for Constipation

Whether it's a continual problem or something that just comes around every now and then, we've all experienced constipation. At any given moment, it will affect over 4.5 million Americans and will send more than 2.5 million of them to their doctors this year alone.

Constipation is a condition in which bowel movements are abnormally delayed, infrequent, and/or incomplete. For many, it's a problem that passes with time or a simple fast. But for millions, chronic constipation is the subtle culprit responsible for many other serious health problems.

In the 20th century there have been few medical topics that have been written about as much as constipation. It is one of many digestive disorders that has plagued Western civilization this century. In fact, constipation, hemorrhoids, ulcerative colitis, irritable bowel syndrome, Crohn's disease, and even appendicitis were rarely seen in the Western world 100 years ago.

This phenomena is still evident today in other non-Westernized nations, like some parts of modern-day Africa, where very little evidence of these disorders is

Help for Inflammatory Bowel Disease

Bowel problems cause more health troubles than most people realize. Having a healthy bowel is usually a good sign of a healthy individual. And now individuals suffering from Inflammatory Bowel Disease (IBD) may have some help in maintaining a healthy bowel.

According to experts at a recent Cleveland Clinic Foundation meeting, vitamin and mineral supplementation is often beneficial for IBD sufferers. "In addition, these patients may have serum levels that indicate no deficiencies of these nutrients. As a result, serum levels should not be relied upon before giving consideration to supplementation in these patients," according to Dr. Joel B. Mason, of the divisions of nutrition and gastroenterology at Tufts University School of Medicine. Dr. Mason is also part of the U.S. Department of Agriculture Human Nutrition Research Center on Aging in Boston.

continued on next page

seen. But the evidence begins to appear as soon as a society takes on the lifestyle of the Western countries.

Diet and Lifestyle

The simple fact that this misery is a product of modern civilization has aided researchers in finding a cure.

Help for Inflammatory Bowel Disease (cont.)

He adds, "Anorexia, restrictive diet, malabsorption due to disease or surgery, diarrhea, bleeding of intestinal mucosa, or drug-nutrient interactions can all have an adverse effect on vitamin and mineral levels in these patients. For example, five to 60 percent of Crohn's disease patients may have low levels of plasma B_{12}. The prevalence of low levels of serum folate is three to 64 percent in hospitalized IBD patients. Also, 25 to 65 percent of these patients may have low levels of 25-hydroxy-vitamin D.

"Prednisone and cholestyramine, two drugs commonly used in these patients, can inhibit the action of vitamin D. IBD patients should receive 200 to 400 IU of vitamin D per day. While iron deficiency is common, oral supplementation frequently causes nausea and vomiting. If the deficiency is greater than 300 mg, parenteral supplementation is recommended." (*Alternative & Complementary Therapies*, October 1994)

They have noticed that the tribespeople in various parts of the earth have a much healthier digestive tract than the peoples of Western civilization. The reason? Their diet is much less opulent than ours. Where we have a tendency to overeat, they usually eat just enough to satisfy their hunger.

"Then there is another reason," says Dr. H.C.A. Vogel, author of *The Nature Doctor*, "The more primitive peoples usually have more fiber in their diet, and this provides the necessary roughage to stimulate the intestinal muscles. We gorge ourselves on white bread, rolls, pastries, puddings, and all kinds of sweets and dishes made from bleached flour and refined sugar, which all contribute to a slowing down of the bowel movement, causing constipation."

Dr. George Meinig, author of *"NEW"trition*, explains why sugar and refined grain foods contribute so heavily to constipation. He says these foods "allow the intestinal contents to build up and pack, much like clay, causing the intestine to swell and become larger in diameter and therefore more difficult to evacuate."

When constipation is due to a diet laden with sugar and refined grains, the most obvious way to correct it is by changing your diet. Eliminate all foods that are generally inclined to promote constipation until the problem has dissipated. These include cheese, eggs and egg dishes, chocolate and all other sugar-rich foods, white bread and other bakery goods made with refined flour, and white rice.

Add to your diet foods that are high in fiber. These include coarse wheat bran, rice bran, and wholegrain breads. It's also important to include all sorts of fruits and vegetables, prunes, figs, dates, and lots of fluids.

Bestselling author Jean Carper says in her new book *Food: Your Miracle Medicine*, "High-fiber foods such as bran and vegetables add bulk, mostly by absorbing and retaining water, producing softer stools that pass through the colon more quickly and gently. The fiber bulks up the stool because much of it is undigested. Fiber's coarse particles also mechanically activate nerve reflexes in the colon wall, triggering bowel movements. Other foods such as coffee and prunes can chemically stimulate the bowel into action. You also need plenty of fluids to keep feces soft." (It should be noted that the caffeine in coffee can contribute to constipation in some people.)

The following fruits have been found to help improve elimination: apples, pears, fresh pineapple, persimmons, figs (fresh and dried), and prunes. For best results, the figs and prunes should not be cooked. Instead, place them in a bowl and pour some boiling water over them. Let them soak overnight and then eat them. If you wish to sweeten them, stir some honey into the boiling water before it is poured.

The importance of diet in relation to constipation is immense. Carper even goes so far as to say that 60 percent of constipation cases can be cleared up simply by adding a little daily bran to the diet. Dr. Alison M. Stephen of the University of Saskatchewan warns that most of us eat about 20 grams of fiber each day, when we should be eating at least twice that amount.

If you have trouble getting enough bran in your diet, try sprinkling a tablespoon of miller's bran on a bowl of cereal every morning. Try this dosage for several days and see what happens. For your problem, this may be too much or too little, so adjust the amount as needed.

If bran has been deficient in your diet for very long, you may experience some stomach discomfort when you start eating it. The bloating and gas should disappear in two or three weeks. To avoid the discomfort, start out with smaller doses and add more fiber as necessary.

Fiber can be added to your diet in any number of creative ways. Following are recipes for two simple soups that are recommended by Dr. Vogel (these should be eaten every morning with a little crispbread or wholegrain bread): "Cook freshly ground whole wheat, a small chopped onion and a crushed clove of garlic in some water. After taking the soup off the stove, add a little finely chopped parsley and a spoonful of pure olive oil.... For stubborn cases, psyllium seed or ground linseed should be added."

The second recipe will often work for those really stubborn cases of constipation. "First, make an herbal infusion. For sensitive people use cassia stick (cassia fistula, also known as purging cassia) tea; for those less sensitive, use senna leaf, senna pod, or some other herbal tea to stimulate the bowel movement. Brew and strain the tea, then for each person add one small raw potato, diced, with the skin. Mix in a teaspoon of bran and one of linseed. Simmer for 15 minutes. If it does not appeal to you, put it through a sieve and drink the liquid.... The effect of this soup on the bowels is astounding and it works when no other laxative does."

The Western Lifestyle

While diet is probably the largest contributing factor to constipation, there are several other elements within the Western lifestyle that promote the problem. The most obvious is the pace with which we live our lives. We tend to be a people of extremes. We are either extremely busy and stressed or extremely sedentary — with both being major causes of constipation.

When we get swept up into the hustle and bustle of the dog-eat-dog world we live in, simple things like a bowel movement can be delayed until a more convenient time. This chaotic lifestyle and failure to pay attention to "the call of nature" can eventually lead to a retarded movement in the bowels. In addition, Dr. Vogel warns, "Restlessness, anxiety, vexation, and constant hurrying affect the sympathetic nervous system," which can aid in the development of spasmodic constipation.

If you live this type of lifestyle and have a problem with constipation, make sure you have a regular time to relieve yourself. Immediately following breakfast is probably the best time. As Dr. Josephus Goodenough stated back in 1904, "Drink liberally of cold water at bedtime and of hot water as soon as you arise. Then attend to nature's calls 'religiously.' Let nothing hinder."

And remember, if you've lived this way for several years, your problem may not clear up overnight. It took you a while to develop the problem and it will probably take a few weeks to reverse it.

Be patient and learn to relax a little. People who are always in a hurry tend to have trouble eliminating. And as the *Dictionary of the Best Tips and Secrets for Better Health* warns, "If you are continually pressed for time, you can disturb your digestive functions permanently."

The other extreme, the sedentary lifestyle, should also be avoided, "because lack of exercise may contribute to constipation," says Dr. Victor Pellicano in the *New Encyclopedia of Common Diseases*. Dr. Pellicano asserts that "many of the same factors associated with varicose veins are seen in cases of constipation, and for that reason, many people have both. On the other hand, primitive people who eat a lot of high-fiber foods and aren't troubled with constipation rarely get varicose veins, either."

Researchers have found that animals, especially horses, usually don't have a problem with constipation unless they are left in small cages or stalls for extended periods of time. The first thing a farmer will do for a constipated animal is exercise it. We can learn a lot from this treatment. If you have a sedentary occupation or lifestyle, a brisk walk in the morning will go a long way toward relief. A morning walk will also help the person whose constipation is due to stress or a busy lifestyle.

Homeopathy and Childhood Diarrhea

"Nicaraguan children under five years old treated with homeopathic remedies stopped having diarrhea two and a half days after starting treatment compared with four days for children who did not receive the remedies, according to a double-blind study conducted by Jennifer Jacobs, M.D., and other researchers at the University of Washington School of Public Health.

"A total of 18 different homeopathic remedies were administered to half of 81 children, including arsenic, chamomile, quicksilver, May-apple, and flowers of sulfur. The children were experiencing diarrhea for less than one week. The remaining half of the children received a placebo. All of the children drank conventional fluid replacement."

Homeopathic remedies can be purchased at most health food stores and many drugstores. (*Pediatrics*, May 1994; *Alternative & Complementary Therapies*, October 1994)

In addition to diet and lifestyle, there are several other factors that need to be considered when searching out a cure for your constipation. The causes of constipation are many, and to find a cure you must find the root cause and treat it. Just treating the symptom of constipation can make the situation worse.

The Problem with Commercial Laxatives

Because of the extreme lifestyles of Western civilization, many people have fallen into the trap of taking commercial laxatives on a regular basis, and are now complaining about spending a small fortune in vain.

As it has for most illnesses, the drug industry in the United States has been quick to provide constipation sufferers with short-cut remedies that fix the symptom and not the main problem. So popular are these quick-fixes that over-the-counter laxatives are now a multi-billion dollar industry.

An excellent example of the quick-fix "syndrome" in America comes from a study reported in the *Journal of the American Geriatric Society*. The study, conducted by a team of researchers from the University of Maryland School of Pharmacy, revealed that laxatives are prescribed more often than any other drug in our nation's nursing homes. The study also showed that very few of the constipated patients in these homes are advised to alter their diet.

On the other hand, researchers at the University of Umea in Sweden found that dramatic results were achieved by adding fiber-rich crispbread (Wasa Fiber) to the diets of their elderly patients. Patricia Hausman and Judith Benn Hurley, authors of *The Healing Foods*, reported that the average patient involved in the study ate five pieces of bread each day and was able to decrease his laxative consumption by 93 percent. (Crispbread can be purchased at most specialty stores.)

The idea behind commercial laxatives is actually quite good, especially for occasional constipation: relax the muscles in the intestine to reduce constriction and allow the blockage to pass. Unfortunately, the means by which the drug industry has gone about accomplishing this have often caused more problems than they solve.

Because of the popular appeal of a quick-fix, commercial laxatives have been overused in the United States. Researchers have discovered that this habit of using laxatives too often will damage your colon and eventually make your constipation problem worse.

In the book *The New Medicine Show*, produced by *Consumer Reports*, further evidence is given to the problems created by laxatives: "Repeated purging in time brings changes in the lining and muscle tone of the bowel; the lining can become irritated and inflamed, and with long-continued catharsis muscular reflexes can become so diminished that stronger and stronger stimulation is required to produce activity. Chronic laxative abusers may also unknowingly be depleting their body of potassium, resulting in muscle weakness. Moreover, many users of cathartics have suffered from fissure of the anus or hemorrhoids. Such ailments often make defecation so painful that the sufferer tends to postpone a visit to the toilet, with the same results as those occurring in a person who is too busy."

In 1975, a Food and Drug Administration advisory panel determined that 25 percent of the 81 ingredients appearing in over-the-counter laxatives were unsafe or ineffective, with another 20 percent needing further study.

Other studies have even shown that commercial laxatives are addictive. But the drug companies aren't about to tell you any of this. After all, there's nothing like creating more business for yourself.

The most important step you can take in dealing with constipation is to stop taking commercial laxatives. If you are guilty of overusing laxatives you might have flushed your system of the beneficial bacteria you need to properly digest your food. But fortunately, we have a remedy: mix some steamed dried apples, honey, and yogurt and eat it daily. The yogurt will help restore the beneficial bacteria to your system and the apples and honey have a mild laxative effect. Sauerkraut, sour pickles, and sour rye bread also promote the growth of healthy bacteria.

Liver Disorders and Constipation

Very few people realize that their constipation may be due to a malfunction of the liver. The liver is one of our most important organs and serves a vital function in the digestion process. When the liver is abused by a poor diet (either overeating or undereating), serious complications can arise. Unfortunately, the liver does not send out warning signals to indicate when trouble might be on the horizon. So learning how to prevent liver trouble before it starts is to our advantage. This can be accomplished by simply eating unrefined, natural foods like brown rice instead of white rice.

You can tell that you have a liver disorder if the sight or smell of fatty or fried food is no longer pleasing.

Dr. Vogel says that "if you cannot tolerate fried potatoes any longer although they used to be a favorite dish, you can be sure that you are suffering from a liver disorder, which will need careful attention. Another symptom of a liver problem is an extreme sensitivity to fruit, for example, oranges or orange juice suddenly upset you.... In this case your liver has lost its ability to digest the fruit acid."

If you are suffering from a liver problem, try eating some walnuts. Walnuts are the only nuts that act as a bowel stimulant. The reason for this effect is that walnuts stimulate the function of the liver which directly influences the bowels.

Another remedy that has been known to work even for severe cases of constipation is an herb tablet called Rasayana No. 2. Rasayana (the Persian name for fennel seed) tablets contain curcuma root and serve to stimulate the liver. If you cannot find Rasayana in your area, it can be ordered from Super Bahar at 404-252-2210.

Acid Deficiency and Constipation

One cause of constipation that is often overlooked, especially in patients over the age of 40, is a condition called hypochlorhydria or achlorhydria (depending on whether your body has little or no stomach acid). After the age of 40, your body's production of hydrochloric acid (HCl) begins to dwindle. If it dwindles enough, you may have trouble digesting meat, fowl, fish, or dairy products. If you lose your taste for meat, you have probably lost the ability to digest it.

Another way to determine if your body is producing enough HCl, according to Dr. Meinig, is to "drink a half glassful of red beet juice and if your urine afterward is colored red it is assumed too little stomach acid was present to digest it. If urine remains yellow it is presumed that sufficient hydrochloric acid was present in the stomach."

If this test reveals an HCl deficiency, Dr. Michael E. Rosenbaum, coauthor of *Super Supplements*, recommends that you take one to three betaine hydrochloride tablets at the beginning of a protein meal. He is also quick to caution that betaine should not be used if you have excess stomach acid or peptic ulcers. Betaine supplements can be purchased at most health food stores. You will probably notice that Dr. Rosenbaum's recommendation is contrary to the directions on the bottle. But don't panic, most doctors agree with his advice.

Other Remedies

If you have a sweet tooth and are looking to satisfy that as well as help your constipation, you might try some blackstrap molasses. Taking one or two tablespoons of molasses before bedtime is a popular remedy in the Balkans, says Lelord Kordel's *Natural Folk Remedies*. "It's also a good source of important minerals, and is rich in the B vitamins, which help fight constipation by toning and strengthening the muscles of the intestinal tract."

Many people don't care for the taste of molasses. If you're one of them, you can stir it into a glass of your favorite beverage (water, milk, juice, etc.). Or, better yet, mix it with a glass of prune juice, for an added laxative benefit.

Kordel also mentions another "concentrated sweet" that has mild laxative properties — honey. This one may be too mild for most cases of constipation, but can be mixed half and half with blackstrap molasses for a stronger dosage.

Linseed

One of the most widely recommended natural laxatives is linseed. This remedy is quite popular with the farmers in Japan and many people in America are singing its praises as well. Linseed has gained its popularity by being one of the most effective foods for regulating the functions of the intestine. It is rich in fiber and contains a substance called mucilage that provides a soothing action and reduces irritation of the intestinal mucous membranes.

You can eat linseed several ways, including raw, sprinkled over salads and cereals, cooked in cereal, or as a liquid mixed in prune, pear, carrot, or apple juice for an added laxative effect. The usual dosage is one tablespoon of whole seeds, two or three times a day, followed by two cups of water. The water will prevent the linseed from causing the formation of lumps on your intestine.

Natural Laxatives

If you have noticed an occasional problem with constipation due to a specific food you've eaten, stress, or some other temporary factor, you might be interested in trying one of the following herbs. These herbs are known to be natural laxatives and will often work for simple cases of constipation. Some, like cascara sagrada, can be effective even for chronic cases.

According to *Rodale's Illustrated Encyclopedia of Herbs*, "Laxatives work by stimulating the peristaltic action of the intestinal wall, by moistening the colon, by increasing the secretion of bile, or by relaxing intestinal cramps."

It should be noted that the body responds to some of these herbs as it does to many of the over-the-counter laxatives. If taken regularly over long periods of time, they can produce dangerous side effects. Therefore, herbs that stimulate the bowel should only be used for the occasional treatment of constipation.

Agar-agar

A mineral-rich gelatine made from seaweed that helps regulate the bowels by forming a smooth, slippery bulk in the intestinal tract. It makes an excellent natural laxative and is easy to use. Simply combine it with fruit juice or fresh fruit to make a gelatine salad or dessert. Or you can use it as a base for soups and puddings. There are several other varieties of seaweed (dulse, wakame, kombu, hiziki) that are sold dry and can easily be added to soups and casseroles. These also have laxative properties that are similar to agar-agar.

Alfalfa

The leaves of the alfalfa plant are an ideal resource for several minerals, nutrients, and amino acids. It is very effective as a laxative, but has been known to aggravate lupus and other autoimmune disorders. According to Earl Mindell's *Herb Bible*, you can take alfalfa orally in several different ways. First, you can take three to six capsules each day. You can also mix one tablespoon of the dried herb with eight ounces of warm water for a daily cup of tea. Finally, you can toss alfalfa sprouts in your favorite salad.

Barberry

The roots of the barberry can be used very effectively to stimulate the smooth muscle of the intestine. The best way to use barberry as a laxative is to prepare an infusion from 1/2 ounce to 1 pint of water. The recommended dosage is 1 to 4 cups daily, taken before meals. Because barberry is so bitter, it should be taken in small doses, a mouthful at a time. Also, 1 tablespoon of a decoction of barberry can be taken as needed.

Basil

This member of the mint family is recommended for many digestive complaints including stomach cramps, gas, vomiting, and constipation. Steep one teaspoon of the dried leaves in a cup of boiling water and enjoy and afterdinner cup of basil tea.

Blue Flag

According to *Dr. Goodenough's Home Cures and Herbal Remedies*, the fresh dried root of blue flag "given in doses of six to eight grains, night and morning, proves gently laxative and eradicates the most inveterate taint of the system.... The leaves in infusion, or a syrup made from the blossoms, is a good medicine for ... loosening the bowels." The plant can be found throughout the United States in the borders of swamps and in wet meadows.

Butternut

Herbalists claim that the inner bark (in powdered form) of the butternut tree is very effective as a mild laxative. In fact, many prefer it over cascara sagrada because it is reputed to not gripe or cramp the intestines like cascara can when used incorrectly.

Cascara Sagrada

Modern science has tried in vain to create a synthetic drug that can duplicate the mild and speedy action of this "sacred bark." However, cascara can now be purchased in the form of pills, powders, and liquids.

According to *Rodale's Illustrated Encyclopedia of Herbs*, "The active ingredients that make cascara such an effective laxative are two types of a substance known as anthraquinone. The first type, free anthraquinone, causes an increased peristalsis, or movement, in the large intestine. The other type, sugar derivative, is absorbed in the digestive tract and circulated through the bloodstream. These sugar derivatives eventually reach a nerve center in the large intestine and trigger a laxative effect."

Using freshly stripped bark is not advised, because it "can cause nausea and a terrible griping effect on the intestinal system. It is best to let the bark sit in storage for one year or to artificially dry the bark at 100 degrees Celcius for one hour. The drying process makes the bark more acceptable to the digestive system. However, unusually large doses or habitual use of the dried bark can have similar effects to those caused by the freshly stripped bark.

You should not use cascara if you suffer from irritable bowel syndrome, ulcers, or are a nursing mother (the laxative effect will be transmitted to your infant).

Dissolving 10 to 30 grains of the store-bought powdered bark extract in water is the recommended dosage of cascara. If you can get your hands on properly dried cascara bark, try the following recipe: Place one teaspoon of bark and 1 1/2 pints of water in a covered con-tainer and slowly boil for about 30 minutes. Remove from the heat and allow the liquid to cool while leaving it covered. A small dose of one tablespoon of the *cold* solution should be taken each day, as needed.

For a mild laxative effect, you might try eating honey that has been made from the cascara flower.

Castor Bean

Castor oil, made from the castor bean, is fairly mild as a laxative and is still widely prescribed for children and elderly patients. Too much of a good thing, though, can bring on nausea and vomiting.

Chicory

Many herbalists consider a decoction of the chicory root to be a mild laxative. Chicory's traditional medicinal property as a laxative is very similar to that of the dandelion.

Dandelion

While the plant is generally regarded as a common lawn pest, the dandelion root has held a distinguished place as an herbal medicine among European herbalists for centuries. The juice of the root is often prescribed as a mild laxative. Or you can take a hot or cold decoction of the root in six-ounce doses three or four times a day. The leaves can also be eaten raw in salads.

Dock

This herb's main medicinal value is as a laxative and is best administered in an infusion. Place one teaspoonful of the dried root in a cup, add boiling water, and steep for 30 minutes. Strain off the root and reheat the tea. Recommended dosage is one or two cups per day.

Fenugreek

Usually, when something is said to cure just about anything under the sun, it won't cure anything. But research suggests that fenugreek may have some medicinal merit. The seeds contain a large amount of mucilage, which may be responsible for fenugreek tea's value as a laxative. Fenugreek tea can be made by steeping one ounce of seeds in one pint of boiling water.

Garlic

You probably know that garlic is great for your health, but few people realize that it also has a stimulating effect on the walls of the stomach and intestine.

Licorice

In this country, licorice powder has been widely used as a mild laxative. It is especially effective for elderly people and children. Up to three inches of the root of the licorice plant can be chewed, as needed. Also, a decoction can be taken in one tablespoon doses, as needed. If you have high blood pressure or use steroid drugs of any kind, you should avoid licorice altogether.

Olive

The oil of the olive promotes contraction of the bowels, so it is an effective laxative. For best results, drink one to two ounces once daily.

Parsley

Parsley leaves are rich in vitamins, including calcium, iron, vitamins A, B, and C. But it's the root of parsley that has laxative properties. According to Gaea and Shandor Weiss, authors of *Growing & Using Healing Herbs*, the root of the parsley plant "is one of five major laxative roots used by European herbalists." These herbalists often use the roots and leaves in a decoction.

Psyllium

Earl Mindell's *Herb Bible* says, "Ground-up seeds from the psyllium plant are one of the highest sources of dietary fiber to be found in any food. For centuries, psyllium has been used to treat ulcers, colitis, and constipation." To use, mix one teaspoon of the ground seeds or powder into one cup of liquid and drink two to three times each day.

Rose

Like parsley, rosehips (the fruit of the plant) are rich in vitamin C and are mildly laxative. Almost all health food stores sell rosehips as a staple.

Know When to See Your Doctor

In most instances, constipation is not a serious malady. However, there are times when a physician should be consulted. If any of the following characteristics describes your case of constipation and the remedies mentioned in this report fail to work, please pay a visit to your doctor.

- Your symptoms have lasted longer than three weeks.
- Stools are thin or "squeezed" (these may be a sign of an obstruction in the bowels).
- If your constipation comes on suddenly and stays longer than usual.

- The problem becomes disabling.
- You find blood in your stool.
- You experience extreme abdominal pain.
- You are vomiting feculent material.
- Your stools show signs of pus or mucous.

Please remember that most cases of constipation are just minor problems and, except for these unusual circumstances, a trip to the doctor should be a rare event.

Chapter 18

Cool Relief From Hemorrhoids

If you have high blood pressure and you're taking one or more of the aforementioned remedies, you might also notice that your hemorrhoids are clearing up. That really shouldn't come as a surprise, especially when you realize that both hypertension and hemorrhoids are often the direct result of a digestive disorder.

Hemorrhoids are basically varicose veins in the lining of the anus. They can occur internally near the beginning of the anus or externally at the opening. Their symptoms include bleeding and protrusion of tissues. They can also cause terrible discomfort and pain during a bowel movement or simply sitting in a chair.

Most treatment programs for hemorrhoids begin with the diet, and rightfully so. If you eat a diet largely made of refined foods that are low in fiber, you're asking for problems. A low-fiber diet will produce small, hard stools that are difficult to pass, resulting in constipation — the number one cause of hemorrhoids. Therefore, the first step in hemorrhoid treatment is to increase the amount of whole fiber foods and raw fruits and vegetables in your diet. (See chapter 17 on constipation.)

But because hemorrhoids are so common in America, we've had to come up with some remedies that are meant specifically for the hemorrhoid, not just the digestive tract. These include everything from suppositories to ointments to herbal teas. The number of treatments for hemorrhoids is voluminous, so we will only address a few simple applications in this chapter.

Pilewort

In Europe, where natural medicine is the rule rather than the exception, hemorrhoid sufferers insist that the aptly named pilewort (or collinsonia in the U.S.) is unmatched among hemorrhoid treatments. According to

---

Another Simple Hemorrhoid Cure

"In your chapter on hemorrhoids, I think you should have mentioned this great remedy: homemade ice suppositories right out of the freezer. Simple to make or use, they can be carved out of an ice cube and work miracles. After only two applications of this process, my wife (who had suffered hemorrhoids for years) has not been bothered since 1989. They seem to have shrunken to nothing. There was some discomfort (cold), but it was well worth it. Thought you would like to know a good remedy!!" — *R.L., Georgia*

Alternative Medicine, the Europeans "combine the tinctures of collinsonia, cranesbill, and ginkgo in equal parts and take one teaspoonful of this mixture three times a day. A topical application is used to alleviate the symptoms and compliment the internal treatment. Mix 10 ml. of collinsonia tincture with 80 ml. of distilled witch hazel and apply this combination after every bowel motion and as needed."

Pilewort can also be used in a tea mixed with equal parts of mullein, yarrow, and wild alum root. Mix the herbs together thoroughly and place one teaspoon in a pint of boiling water. Let boil and then steep for 30 minutes. Drink half a cup three or four times daily.

Glycerine Suppositories

According to Jethro Kloss, author of *Back to Eden*, "The following is a very excellent remedy for healing when used as a suppository:

2 ounces powdered hemlock bark

1 ounce golden seal

1 ounce powdered wheat flour

1 ounce boric acid

1 ounce bayberry bark

"Mix with glycerine until it is stiff enough to form suppositories. Insert one into the rectum at night and leave it in place."

A slight variation of this glycerine suppository that also works is made with black mullein, calendula, comfrey, plantain, or slippery elm bark.

Comfrey powder can also be mixed with water to form a paste or with petroleum jelly to form an excellent ointment.

Apple Cider Vinegar

Apple cider vinegar taken internally and used topically has been a popular remedy for years. In her book *Treasury of Home Remedies*, Myra Cameron gives several uses for apple cider vinegar: "The Vermont folk remedy for chronic hemorrhoids is to stir two teaspoons each apple cider vinegar and honey in a glass of water to sip with each meal. A variation said to stop any itching and make the piles vanish in three weeks is to stir one teaspoon of the vinegar in the glass of water to drink with each meal and to use another glass of the same mixture for daily external applications. Annoying itching may be relieved by saturating a cotton ball with apple cider vinegar and inserting it overnight."

Hot and Cold Applications

Alternating hot and cold applications will do wonders for your circulation and for the most painful hemorrhoids. The easiest method is to use two hand towels or washcloths, one soaked in hot water, the other in cold. After wringing out the excess water, place the hot towel on the hemorrhoid for three minutes. Then replace it with the cold towel. After 30 seconds, reheat the hot towel, if necessary, and place it on the hemorrhoid. Continue this process for 30 minutes.

You can also do this method by taking a hot sitz bath for at least 15 minutes and then sitting in a cold bath (already prepared) for a minute or two. Then return to the hot bath (reheated, if necessary) and repeat the process for one hour. This method is not as convenient as the towel method, but is usually more effective.

But My Doctor Says ...

Many times a doctor will tell you that your hemorrhoid must be surgically removed. But as you have now seen, a good natural treatment will usually address the problem much better and with fewer (if any) complications or side effects. Before submitting to surgery, make sure you've exhausted all other avenues of treatment. Your body will thank you for it in the long run.

Chapter 19

Heartburn: The Fire Within

You've just returned home from a wonderful dinner at your favorite Italian restaurant and are looking forward to a relaxing evening in front of the TV. Then it hits. That awful burning sensation in your chest that ruins any thoughts of relaxation.

The problem is heartburn, and in this case it's caused by acid reflux. Most people experience it when they gorge themselves at the dinner table. Over-filling the stomach forces some of the stomach juices out of the stomach and back up the esophagus (the pipe that runs between your mouth and stomach). Included among these juices is hydrochloric acid (HCl), and if you've ever taken a chemistry class you know that HCl is a highly corrosive substance. Fortunately, your stomach has a lining that protects the organ from the destructive properties of HCl, but your esophagus doesn't provide that luxury. Thus, the burning sensation.

While acid reflux is usually responsible for the pain, Jane Heimlich, associate editor of *Health & Healing* and author of *What Your Doctor Won't Tell You*, says that too much acid is not always the cause: "After age 40, production of HCl dwindles ... so if you don't have enough, you may have trouble digesting meat, fowl, fish, or dairy products.... To determine if you need HCl, James F. Balch, M.D., coauthor of *Prescription for Nutritional Healing* ... suggests this simple test: When experiencing heartburn, take a tablespoon of apple cider vinegar or lemon juice. If this relieves your symptoms, then you need more HCl; if the symptoms become worse ... you have too much HCl.

"If you need HCl, Michael E. Rosenbaum, M.D., coauthor of *Super Supplements*, recommends taking one to three betaine hydrochloride tablets at the beginning of a protein meal.... Caution: Betaine is not recommended for persons with excess stomach acid or peptic ulcers.

"All betaine products sold in health food stores are similar.... Note: Directions on betaine products are contrary to Dr. Rosenbaum's recommendation. I have

---

A Honey of a Cure

"When my wife or I feel a little stomach upset, bilious, or nauseated, a teaspoonful of honey usually gives us quick relief. When we travel honey is an item we carry in our luggage and several times when we became ill or another party in our tour group became ill, honey *saved the day*! I believe honey has been reported to kill several kinds of bacteria." — *J.M.A., California*

consulted other doctors, and they agree with Dr. Rosenbaum's prescription."

If, however, you find that you do have an over-abundance of HCl, you might try some of the following simple remedies. If none of these remedies relieve your pain, you may have a more serious problem. You may have an ulcer, intestinal worms, or a dysfunction in your gallbladder.

The Daily Blaze

Ten percent of the American population suffers from heartburn on a daily basis. For these people, heartburn could have some serious complications. These complications may include coughing, bronchitis, pneumonitis, asthma, bleeding in the esophageal lining (leading to anemia), and constriction of the esophagus tube (making swallowing difficult).

Chronic heartburn almost always occurs when the lower esophageal sphincter (LES — the muscle at the junction of the esophagus and the stomach) weakens or relaxes, allowing the gastric juices to flow into the esophagus. Most of the time, this is caused by certain foods in the diet that cause the LES to relax. Avoiding spicy, acidic, fatty, or tomato-based foods, coffee, alcohol, carbonated drinks, chocolate, and mints will usually be enough to fix the problem.

Also, if you are suffering from heartburn and are on any prescription drug, you should talk to your doctor. A number of prescription drugs, including some antidepressants and sedatives, may aggravate heartburn.

Antacids Work, But ...

If you suffer from a really stubborn case of heartburn, don't bother listening to the antacid commercials on TV. Many of the popular antacids contain aluminum, a substance that has been linked to Alzheimer's disease and should be avoided at all costs. Long-term use of antacids, according to Dr. William Stern of George Washington University School of Medicine, can also cause constipation or diarrhea, depending on the brand and its ingredients.

Dr. Herta Spencer of the Veterans Administration Hospital in Hines, Illinois, said in *The Dictionary of Medical Folklore* that, taken daily, even low doses of some of the antacids can affect the body's ability to metabolize phosphorus and calcium. The result may be general body weakness, some pain, a loss of appetite, and, eventually, a weakening of the bones.

Try Some Potato Juice

There are those cases of heartburn that may require the professional help of a doctor. But before you spend $50 on a doctor's visit and $25 on the subsequent prescription, you might try some of the following advice:

Dr. H.C.A. Vogel, author of *The Nature Doctor*, says that "A number of simple remedies exist for heartburn.... All you need do first is to grate a [raw] potato as finely as possible, then put this in a cheesecloth and press out the juice. Dilute with warm water, one part juice to two or three parts water. Drink this juice every morning before breakfast, before lunch, and at night before retiring. For best results, prepare fresh each time."

Wood Ash and Charcoal

If the fire in your chest is still burning, Dr. Vogel recommends that you "take a teaspoon of wood ash mixed in a little warm water after eating.... Just pour warm water over the ashes and drink them down. If you have no wood ash, common charcoal, preferably from limewood, can be crushed and mixed with a little water, porridge, or other cereal. The charcoal is easier to swallow when prepared in this way and will serve to neutralize the stomach acid. If you do not find the idea of taking wood ash as described above appealing, pour hot water over them and brew in the same way you would make a pot of tea, straining through a fine sieve or cheesecloth. This liquid will also neutralize the gastric acid. Clay (white or yellow) dissolved in a little water is equally effective." And if you can't see yourself eating common charcoal, activated charcoal tablets are available at health food stores.

Dr. Vogel also mentions that "sipping fresh milk will give temporary relief." This has been a popular recommendation for years. However, there is a problem with milk. The fats, proteins, and calcium in milk will cause the stomach to secrete acid. So the temporary relief you get from the milk going down will be just that — temporary.

Herbal Remedies

Many herbal treatments have also been suggested for heartburn. Some herbalists maintain that the juices of Betony can be effectively used. *Rodale's Illustrated Encyclopedia of Herbs* indicates that a decoction of Fenugreek taken a cup at a time, three times a day, will work. Dr. Daniel B. Mowrey, a psychologist and psychopharmacologist who has been researching herb use in medicine for 15 years, said in *The Doctors Book of Home Remedies* that gingerroot is the most helpful. "I've seen it work often enough that I'm convinced." Start by taking two capsules just before you eat and increase the dosage as you need to. Dr. Mowrey says that you've taken enough when you start to taste ginger in your throat.

Dr. Mowrey also indicates that the class of herbs called bitters (e.g., gentian root, wormwood, and goldenseal) is also helpful when taken in capsule form or as a liquid extract.

The Nutritional Approach

Nutrition experts Harvey and Marilyn Diamond offer a different approach in their book *Fit for Life*: "If you want to have a steak, or a piece of fish or chicken, so be it. Just be aware that if you're going to have any flesh food, that is your one concentrated food for *that* meal. That means with it you should not have any other concentrated foods. Not potatoes, rice, noodles, cheese, or bread, but with it have high-water-content food. In other words, along with the steak have some vegetables.... It can be any vegetable you like. Understand that vegetables do not need their own specific digestive juices. They will break down in either medium, acid, or alkaline."

The Diamonds' approach calls for a simple diet that should be heeded by anyone who suffers from serious heartburn. Eating simply puts less stress on your stomach and digestive system. It also allows you to enjoy the foods you love to eat, just not all at the same time.

Conclusion

The two most important points to remember about heartburn are: (1) it's just a symptom of a problem, not the real problem, and (2) the problem is almost always related to diet. This means there is good news and bad news connected to heartburn. The good news is that it can usually be fixed without a trip to the doctor. The bad news, though, is that it may take some dietary changes, which means you must employ the dreaded "D" word — Discipline. But if you can manage it, you'll save your body from a world of damage.

Chapter 20

Questions and Answers

Ulcers

Q. I've been suffering from ulcers for years and have been unable to get rid of them. My doctor wants to prescribe antibiotics, but I'd prefer to use a natural remedy. Are there any?

A. For chronic ulcers you might want to try taking a tablespoon of aloe vera gel. The Newsletter of Advanced Natural Therapies suggests that during the most virulent attacks you take this dosage every hour. Once you are out of the critical stage "you can take from one to two tablespoons of aloe vera three or four times a day until the ulcers are completely healed. According to one researcher, aloe vera gives the fastest and most permanent relief of any substance he has seen."

The concentrate made from the aloe plant is also very effective for other digestive and colonic problems. Several whole-leaf aloe products are sold in most health food stores. But be warned, don't try to make the gel on your own; if it's not prepared properly it can cause a severe case of diarrhea. And of course, you don't want to take aloe if you're allergic to it.

Bladder Infections

Q. I realize that women often suffer from bladder infections, but I never had any such trouble until I got married. Why is that? And what can I do about it?

A. There are certain times in a woman's life when bladder infections (cystitis) tend to flare up with a certain degree of predictability. It just so happens that flare-ups during the honeymoon are so common that the problem has been called "honeymoon cystitis." The reason for this is not certain, but according to the *New Encyclopedia of Common Diseases*, many researchers theorize "that any bacteria in the neighborhood of the urethra have a good chance of being pushed up into the bladder during intercourse."

Unfortunately, the problem doesn't always end when the honey-moon is over. Studies show that 80 percent of women with a history of cystitis will suffer from the problem again, most likely during pregnancy. This means you need a non-toxic way to fight the infection.

New studies are now confirming that cranberry juice is an effective treatment for bladder infections. The *Journal of the American Medical Association* reported in the March 9, 1994 issue that the ingestion of cranberry juice reduces the frequency of infection. Dr. Jerry Avorn, associate professor of medicine, Harvard Medical School, said, "There's a substance in cranberries and blueberries that may prevent the adhesiveness of bacteria to the bladder wall."

Incontinence

Q. My husband has a terrible problem with incontinence, but is so embarrassed by it that he won't see a doctor or even talk about it. It's gotten so bad that he won't leave the house. Is there anything I can do that will help him? It's really taking the life out of our marriage.

A. As a matter of fact, there is something you can do to help your husband's problem. Incontinence is not a life-threatening problem, but it is terribly humiliating. And it can have terrible implications for people who are very active socially.

Ironically, when you find yourself urinating too frequently, you need an herb that makes you urinate, like parsley. But Sam Biser, editor of *Advanced Natural Therapies* newsletter, says that you also need other herbs like juniper berries, uva ursi, black cohosh, marshmallow root, gingerroot, lobelia, gravel root, and white pond lily. "You can make a formula yourself with equal parts of the herbs," writes Biser, "and drink two to three glasses of this tea each day. (Use one to two teaspoons of herbs per glass of tea.)" You can buy each of these individual herbs from your local herb shop or health food store.

Weak Stomach

Q. I have a serious problem with my stomach. After eating a meal, the food seems to sit like a rock for hours — almost like I can't digest it. I've tried all the antacids, but they don't work. Is there something wrong with me, or is it the food I'm eating, or both? I also have heart problems and I've heard that the two problems could be linked. Is this possible?

A. It is true that many health problems are caused by our diet. Whether your heart problems are linked to your digestive problems is hard to tell (it could be genetic), but it is definitely possible.

As far as your weak stomach is concerned, Mannfried Pahlow gives an ironic twist to gastrointestinal problems in his book, *Healing Plants*. He says the use of hearty seasonings is often better for digestive problems than the normally prescribed bland diet.

He says, "Long ago it was scientifically proved that herbs and spices can stimulate the appetite or make the digestion of food easier, because they activate the glands that produce gastric juice. In addition, they can lessen the strain on the heart and circulatory system.

"Spicy seasonings in particular intensify the progress of almost all vital processes, which results in increased vitality. If you want an all-around feeling of well-being, frequently add spicy seasonings like paprika, cayenne pepper, ginger, mustard, or turmeric to your foods....

"In Mexico, where people enjoy eating fiery chili peppers, and in the Balkans, where hot paprika is popular, fewer people suffer heart attacks than in this country. As research over time has revealed, the spices used are partially responsible.

"Before the positive effect of seasonings on our health could be proved, it was considered nutritionally incorrect for older people or people with gastrointestinal problems to season their foods heartily — a bland diet was recommended. The opposite is true, however...."

For a weak stomach, the herbs that Pahlow recommends you use frequently as seasonings include: mugwort, wormwood, basil, summer savory, marjoram, and thyme. Mustard, paprika, nutmeg, ginger, and hot curry have also proved to be beneficial. "For this purpose," says Pahlow, "the amount of seasoning that suits your taste is usually sufficient."

Hemorrhoids

Q. I've never been one to suffer from hemorrhoids except during pregnancy. However, I just noticed the other day that something has caused them to flare up. So far they have not thrombosed and I'd really like to get rid of them before they get any worse. Do you have any suggestions?

A. There are a number of home remedies that will work for hemorrhoids, especially if you catch them in the early stages. The following testimony from *Natural Home Remedies* is just one example of what can be used.

"Years ago, when my children were small and there was no extra money for large doctors' bills, I developed a bad case of painful and bleeding hemorrhoids.

"The doctor told me the best thing would be an operation. Having to support three lively boys, this shook me up. Money could not stretch for operations. I couldn't take the time off from work. I couldn't afford a babysitter, and the doctor read from my face that it would not do.

"So he told me to go to the drugstore, get a small bottle of witch hazel, prepare a basin of warm water, put

---

Try the Liver Flush Before Gallbladder Surgery

Dr. Nicholas Gonzales of New York says, "The liver flush is just a very simple way of getting rid of gallstones and stored wastes in the gallbladder...."

First, buy a "two-ounce bottle of ortho-phosphoric acid, available in health food stores.... Dump that two-ounce bottle into a gallon of apple juice, shake it up, and drink it down over about a three or four day period, three or four glasses a day. The day you finish the apple juice, there's a series of things you have to do.

"Eat a normal breakfast and a normal lunch, then two hours after lunch take two tablespoons of Epsom salts in a glass of water. Five hours after lunch, take another tablespoon of Epsom salts. Epsom salts is magnesium sulfate and causes diarrhea, but it also relaxes all the ducts that carry waste out of the liver and gallbladder. Normally those are tightly closed. Epsom salts opens them wide to allow stones and bile to pass through.

continued on the next page

Try the Liver Flush Before Gallbladder Surgery (cont.)

"The ortho-phosphate softens and dissolves a lot of these gallstones, and the magnesium sulfate (Epsom salts) taken the last day relaxes the gallbladder duct so it opens wide. For dinner that night you have nothing but fruit in heavy cream, which starts stimulating contraction of the gallbladder.

"Before you go to bed — it sounds awful — you drink half a cup of olive oil on an empty stomach. Olive oil is pure fat. When it hits the stomach, the gallbladder and the liver duct start vigorously contracting and all the stones and the waste material are squeezed right into the intestines. The Epsom salts opens up the ducts, the ortho-phosphate has softened the stones, so when you drink the oil the gallbladder contracts, squirting all that junk into the intestines." (*Moneychanger*, August 1991)

---

a quarter cup of the liquid into the water, and sit in it as long as possible. And to do this whenever possible.

"I did, and before three days had passed, I had not only relief from the itch and pain, but the bleeding had stopped. I kept this up until all symptoms vanished. And, although that was 40 years ago, I've had no pains since."
— *A.G., Pennsylvania*

Ulcerative Colitis

Q. My wife suffers with a diagnosis of ulcerative colitis. My constant reading has yet to agree with what her doctors have prescribed — without any remedy, I might add. She is taking an anti-inflammatory Asacol. My suggestions of dietary restraints and supplements are received as heresy. Can you comment?

A. Many alternative health practitioners agree that the treatment of ulcerative colitis is best handled with proper dietary regulation. Ulcerative colitis and Crohn's disease are the two major categories of inflammatory bowel disease (IBD) and the role of food allergies in chronic inflammatory disease has been well documented.

Most mainstream doctors treat ulcerative colitis with corticosteroids or surgery. The drugs are known to be very harsh and can impair the immune system, while surgery is often ineffective and has many undesirable side effects. Because of these facts, treatment that includes the elimination of allergy-causing foods should be used before the drugs and surgery are considered. Common allergenic foods are wheat, corn, dairy products, and processed foods that contain stabilizers and suspending agents.

Dr. Patrick Donovan of Seattle, Washington, says that in the active phase, a liquid diet consisting of cabbage juice and other green leafy vegetable juices should be used. He also recommends vegetable broths and broths from the seaweeds *wakame, hijiki,* and *kombu.* "Vegetables are then gradually added back into the diet, then blended fruit juices. This is followed by the introduction of meat and fish broths, then solid fish. When patients are back to normal, they can add in animal proteins, grains, and beans."

According to *Alternative Health*, "A patient with a history of colitis for 10 years and no relief from conventional therapy came to Dr. Donovan. He fasted the patient for four days and then put him on vegetable juices and lamb bone broth, after having determined which foods he was allergic to. His iron-deficiency anemia was treated with iron-containing herbs and foods such as spinach and kale. His symptoms began to resolve.

"Over the next 10 days he was put on raw and steamed vegetables and salads, and by the end of a month he was back on a whole foods vegetarian diet. Within 30 days he was able to return to work.

"Supplements of magnesium, calcium, iron, potassium, and multivitamins are needed to counteract the decreased food intake and decreased absorption from the small intestine."

Inflammatory conditions, like ulcerative colitis, often respond well to vegetarian diets. But it's also important to consume plenty of cold-water fish, such as mackerel, herring, sardines, and salmon. Consuming these fish or fish oil supplements significantly reduces the inflammatory/allergic response and has a therapeutic effect on ulcerative colitis. Fish oil supplementation is not necessary if you consume at least one serving of fish every day.

Myasthenia Gravis

Q. Have you any information on how to remedy myasthenia gravis apart from the conventional treatment with Mestinon?

A. Myasthenia gravis is a disease of progressive muscle weakness associated with low gastric acidity (low stomach-acid production). While not a cure, myasthenia gravis is best treated with hydrochloric acid supplementation, which is usually advised to be taken under the supervision of a doctor. However, Dr. Michael T. Murray, author of *Natural Alternatives to Over-the-Counter and Prescription Drugs*, has published a protocol for hydrochloric acid supplementation. It is as follows:

"1. Begin by taking one tablet or capsule containing 10 grains (600 milligrams) of hydrochloric acid (HCl) at your next large meal. If this does not aggravate your symptoms, at every meal of comparable size take one additional tablet or capsule. (One at the next meal; two at the meal after that; three at the next meal.)

"2. Continue to increase the dose until you reach seven tablets, or when you feel a warmth in your stomach — whichever occurs first. A feeling of warmth in the stomach means that you have taken too many tablets for that meal, and you need to take one tablet less for that meal size. It is a good idea to try the larger dose again at another meal to make sure that it was the HCl that caused the warmth and not something else.

"3. After you have found what the largest dose is that you can take at your large meals without feeling any warmth, maintain that dose at all meals of similar size. You will need to take fewer tablets at smaller meals.

"4. When taking a number of tablets or capsules, it is best to space them throughout the meal, rather than taking them all at once.

"5. As your stomach begins to regain the ability to produce the amount of HCl needed to digest your food properly, you will notice the warm feeling again, and will have to cut down the dose level."

Other supplements have also been found to be effective treatments for myasthenia gravis. These include choline, pantothenate, thiamine (B_1), and manganese.

Section 6

Miscellaneous
Health Problems

Chapter 21

Bilberry and Antioxidants Block Cataracts

There are approximately 50 million people around the world suffering from cataracts, a buildup of protein on the eye lens that causes foggy and blurred vision and many times blindness. In fact, the World Health Organization says that half the cases of blindness in the world are caused by cataracts.

What's worse, if you're an unfortunate cataract sufferer, your doctor will probably recommend surgery, as this is conventional medicine's standard treatment. But before you submit your delicate eyes to the hands of a surgeon, you might want to consider some new scientific evidence indicating home remedies might solve your problem.

The Italians have done extensive research on the amazing benefits of bilberry for the eyes. Their studies indicate that persons taking bilberry on a consistent basis have found an average improvement in vision of an astounding 80 percent. One German ophthalmologist said many of his patients were helped by a combination of bilberry extract and dandelion flowers.

Exercise Helps Work Off Glaucoma

"Yet another reason to exercise early and often: Vigorous aerobic workouts relieve the condition that results in glaucoma.

"A leading cause of blindness, glaucoma offers no early-warning signs as it develops. A drainage malfunction inside the eye allows the fluid there, called aqueous humor, to build up. The resulting pressure on the eye eventually leads to permanent vision loss.

"Researchers in Oregon measured the intraocular eye pressure of nine sedentary people suspected of having glaucoma. The people then were put on a three-month program of fairly vigorous exercise that required them to ride a stationary bicycle for 40 minutes four times a week at 70 to 85 percent of their maximum heart rates.

"By the end of the study, the average intraocular pressure had fallen by 20 percent. Three weeks after the exercise program ended, the inside-the-eye pressure had returned to pre-exercise levels.

"Further proof of exercise's influence on the cause of glaucoma came from Finnish researchers who studied people with no indication of the eye disorder. Of four people in the study who had eye pressure significantly above normal, three were able to lower the reading to a normal range through exercise.

"Glaucoma also may respond to nutrition. Many people with the disorder often have deficiencies of chromium and vitamin C, according to Columbia University optometrist Ben C. Lane. I recommend five grams of vitamin C and 400 mcg of chromium (picolinate or nicotinate) every day." (*Dr. Atkins' Health Revelations*, February 1995)

According to John Heinerman, author of *Heinerman's Encyclopedia of Nuts, Berries, and Seeds*, another Italian scientist reported "that when vitamin E (600 IU) and bilberry extract (three capsules) were both taken orally, once a day, they stopped the progression of cataract formation in 97 percent of subjects tested." (*Ann. Ottalmol. Clin. Ocul.*, 115:109, 1989)

The therapeutic value of vitamin E and other antioxidants for the eyes has been documented extensively. Dr. J. Robertson reported in the *American Journal of Nutrition* that "consumption of supplementary vitamin C and E may reduce the risk of senile cataracts by about 50 to 70 percent."

Other evidence shows that cataracts may even be reversed using antioxidants. Why are antioxidants so effective? There is significant data demonstrating the role of free radicals in cataracts. A study reported in *Prevention* magazine "involving 832 people showed that those with the highest blood levels of vitamin E had the fewest cataracts. According to Susan Vitale, assistant professor of ophthalmology at Johns Hopkins University, the risk of cataracts was about cut in half in those people who had the highest blood levels of vitamin E."

The *British Medical Journal* (8/92) published a large-scale study conducted by the Brigham and Women's Hospital and Harvard Medical School. The study found that there is a 40 percent lower rate of cataracts among people who consumed large amounts of food high in vitamin A. The researchers also found that long-term vitamin C supplementation lowered the risk of cataracts.

And finally, the first study ever to link fruit and vegetable consumption to cataracts was reported in the *American Journal of Clinical Nutrition* (January 1991).

According to *Prevention* magazine, the study "showed that people who eat three and a half servings of fruits and vegetables every day have a substantially reduced risk of cataracts. Those who consume less than that are believed to be almost six times more at risk for cataracts than those who do eat these foods, which contain vitamin C and beta carotene."

These are just a few of the abundant studies linking bilberry and antioxidant consumption with a decreased risk of developing cataracts. If you want to protect yourself from cataracts, your best bet is to consume plenty of fresh fruits and vegetables — at least five servings a day. Many new studies are showing that supplements don't appear to have the same effect.

Also, quit smoking. Twenty percent of cataracts are caused by cigarette smoking.

Chapter 22

Skin Ailments and Injuries

Few of us have trouble remembering the days of adolescence when a pimple on the end of your nose was the beginning of the end of life as you knew it. For boys, it meant hearing the girls in your class giggling and the boys cackling. Even your own mother wasn't very sympathetic. She probably said, "I told you not to eat that chocolate bar!"

Well, it probably wasn't the chocolate bar that brought about your dismal situation, but rather, your diet in general. Food has long been known to be a major contributor to this skin affliction. But what most people don't realize is that certain foods can be used effectively as topical treatments.

The most important step to an acne-free complexion is hygiene. Instead of washing your face with soap and water, try using milk or diluted lemon juice; a solution of one part alcohol to 10 parts warm water can also be effective. After using one of these washes, thoroughly rinse the face with warm water and then pat dry. Don't rub vigorously.

Myra Cameron, author of *Treasury of Home Remedies*, says, "Washing with buttermilk and blotting the face

With Athlete's Foot, Less Is More

A new study conducted by Mary-Margaret Chren, M.D., indicates that the less expensive over-the-counter medications are often more effective than the expensive prescription drugs for treating athlete's foot. The study compared miconazole and two other over-the-counter medicines with seven topical creams sold by prescription.

Chren, a dermatologist at the Cleveland Veterans Affairs Medical Center and Case Western Reserve University School of Medicine, said that when taking prescription drugs, "We're operating under the delusion that doctors have the data to support the choices they make. In fact, a doctor's choice is often not bolstered by data."

Chren added, "It's often argued that more expensive drugs are less expensive in the long run. We found that in the long-run it's always cheaper to start with the cheapest drug."

A four-week supply of miconazole cost approximately $9.04. The other eight medications ranged in price from $34.67 to $174.39 for a similar course of treatment.

Doctor's have been avoiding the use of natural treatments for years because the products are not backed by research. Now we find that this argument is baseless. If Chren's comment about your doctor's lack of data to support his prescriptions is true (and we believe it is), why not try a non-drug treatment that's even less expensive than the over-the-counter drug. Tea tree oil has a strong reputation for fighting fungus and it can often be found for less than $8 an ounce. (*Journal of the American Medical Association*, 12/28/94, *Wall Street Journal*, 12/28/94)

That Nasty Poison Ivy

This past summer I was rummaging around in the woods and found my way into a nice patch of poison ivy. Before I knew it, I had blisters forming all over the place; eyes, ears, hands, arms, legs, you name it, it was covered. So naturally, I went looking for relief.

I didn't realize at the time that if I would have taken a few moist "towelettes" with me and wiped the exposed areas of my body with them every 30 minutes, I would have saved myself a load of grief.

Here's why: "Dr. David Harris, a Stanford University dermatologist, suggests if people wipe exposed skin every half-hour with towelettes, they will be wiping off the resin that causes the itchy rash. Research shows that the resin starts binding to the skin within 10 minutes, but up until a half-hour the resin can still be rubbed off with a mild detergent, the same ingredient present in towelettes.

"After a half-hour, however, the poison will have taken a firm hold and it is time to seek follow-up treatments." (*Let's Live*, October 1994)

without rinsing was an old folk remedy, as was rubbing the affected area with lemon juice or fresh garlic several times a day to speed the healing of existing pimples. Warm, double-strength papaya-mint tea has been used as an emergency treatment for acne eruptions."

More Relief From Poison Ivy

"I was a sufferer of poison ivy with truly horrid cases till I discovered the natural wonders of jewel weed. At the first sign of the wicked itch, rubbing the leaf and/or stem on the spots starts it healing. Now I keep a supply of ice cubes made by boiling the leaves and stems of jewel weed in water and then freezing the liquid. Each cube becomes an easy to apply remedy. Jewel weed, which is common around the country, is sometimes called "Touch-me-not" because its small yellow flower pops off so easily." — *R.L.B., New York*

Cameron says there are several other foods that can be used as facial masques, including carrots, cucumber, egg yolk, and oatmeal. Here are four suggestions:

Carrots — Cook in as little water as possible, then mash and apply when comfortably cool. Rinse with lukewarm water after 30 minutes.

Cucumber — Peel if coated with wax. Slice very thin and soak in rum, or simply grate before applying.

Egg Yolk — Whisk and pat over the skin.

Oatmeal — Cook in milk until thickened, then cool and apply.

Another treatment is to apply a bentonite clay facial mask and leave on for 15-20 minutes; rinse off. Apply three times a week.

Turnips and cabbage also make excellent compresses to treat acne. All you have to do is steam them and apply

---

An Udderly Magnificent
Anti-Aging Cream

"A friend in her late 60s has gorgeous, young skin. Her secret is a veterinary product for cow udders called Bag Balm. She used it for 10 years — one application about every 30 to 60 days as a night cream, no soap, only water or shampoo in between.

"Other friends use it for psoriasis, rough hands and feet, and for healing scrapes and bruises. It is inexpensive, can be obtained at veterinary supply stores or at the large chain drugstores.

"It stinks, but it's worth it." — *E.C.H., California*

---

while comfortably warm.

And finally, after you have washed and dried your face, apply the oil from a vitamin E capsule and let it remain for 30 minutes. Then apply a coating of lightly whisked egg white over the vitamin E. Leave this on for another 30 minutes and rinse with filtered water.

There are many other ways to treat acne, but when food is a major cause of the problem, why not use food to solve it? Of course, if serious acne persists, you'll probably have to make dietary adjustments as well as take some vitamin and mineral supplements.

Say What?!?!

"I recently read about a European salve the FDA wanted off the market because it contained animal urine. It was used for cuts, scrapes, and burns. Then I remembered an elderly aunt who used children's wet diapers on their rashes, insect stings, cuts, and burns.

"So the next time I burned my fingers on a hot pan, I tried my own urine. The burn pain increased because of the warmth of the fluid, but dissipated almost immediately. The expected blister never appeared at all!

"I told a friend, and she laughed and said her sons recovered from chronic athlete's foot when their paternal grandpa told them to 'pee' on their feet before they got out of the shower. That put 'paid' to all those over-the-counter remedies in their household.

"My daughter got a silly grin when she heard this and said she'd never had athlete's foot, even when surrounded by those who did, maybe because of an automatic bladder reaction to showers.

"I hope you enjoy my tales herein as much as I enjoyed writing them. Maybe someone else can benefit from them." — *E.C.H., California*

Treating Burns

Identify the Burn

Most burns can be treated at home, but third-degree burns require immediate medical attention. Here's how to tell how badly you are burned:

■ **First-degree** burns are red, slightly swollen, and painful. They include most sunburns and scalds. The only treatment that might be necessary is for the pain as healing usually takes only five to 10 days. Generally, first-degree burns do not leave scars.

■ **Second-degree** burns will blister and ooze and are extremely painful. They are usually caused by extended exposure to the sun and brief contact with oven coils. These burns can usually be treated with simple remedies you can administer at home and will take about 20 days to heal. Second-degree burns can leave scars, but many of the remedies listed below will reduce the scarring.

■ **Third-degree** burns are charred and can be bleached white and dry or brown and calcified. Third degree burns

---

Fast Relief From Cuts and Scrapes

"One of my favorite home remedies for cuts and scrapes is to cut a raw potato in half and rub the inside of it on the cut. The potato will absorb the blood and you will hardly be able to see the cut line. Eggplant also works well in that regard." — *C.S., Ohio*

A Simple Burn Remedy

"I am writing you concerning a remedy from my grandfather. It is Iodoform (CHI3) applied to broken burn blisters. It is a yellow powder that acts as a disinfectant, styptic, and local anesthetic. I understand this was popular a century ago, but a one-ounce bottle I bought about 10 years ago (the smallest available from a pharmacist — without a prescription) bears this warning: Harmful if absorbed through skin. I don't know anyone who has had a bad reaction from it, but that one-ounce bottle should be enough to last several lifetimes for anyone but a blacksmith." — *L.A., Maryland*

destroy the nerve ends, so there is usually no pain. The flesh under the skin is also destroyed and will probably require a skin transplant.

Seek medical care immediately as severe complications can occur. Before you leave for the hospital, though, flush the burn with cold water and then apply unprocessed honey, aloe vera, or vitamin E oil. This will help soothe the pain and could reduce the amount of scarring that takes place. Also, if any clothing is stuck to the burn, do not try to remove it. Let the doctor worry about that.

Listed below are several remedies that will usually work in the treatment of most burns:

Cold Water & Honey

Flushing your burn with lots of cold water will stop the burning. Once you've put out the fire, the healing process can begin. After you've flushed the burn, smother the burn with honey and wrap it in a towel.

Aloe Vera

Growing an aloe vera plant (also know as the "burn plant") in your home is a great way to have a first-aid kit handy for treating burns. When that unfortunate accident occurs simply cut one of the leaves open and apply the jelly directly on the burn. The jelly acts as a disinfectant and anaesthetic and helps restore the skin's natural pigmentation.

Clay

Place a piece of gauze over the wound and apply a half inch clay compress over the gauze for one hour. Change the compress every two hours until new tissue is formed. Then you can reduce the applications to two to four times a day. You can also immerse a burned hand or foot into a mud bath of clay for an hour or two.

Plantain Leaves

Rub the leaves of this plant between your hands until the juice seeps out. Then simply apply the juice to the burn.

Mustard

"My neighbor was cleaning a very, very hot restaurant grill with a block that broke, causing her to scrape both hands right across that blistering hot grill. She was standing there looking at her badly burned hands when a truck driver who had just come into the restaurant yelled at her to put mustard on her hands. She could hardly believe it, but she put her hands right into the large mustard jar near the grill. The pain ceased and she doesn't have a single scar on her hands!" — Iorez W., a subscriber to the newsletter *Alternatives*.

Vitamin E

Simply puncture and squeeze the oil from some alpha-tocopherol vitamin E capsules into a jar of petroleum jelly and apply to burns. Also, take two hundred units of vitamin E capsules orally.

Hydrogen Peroxide

If the burn is on your hands or feet, soak the burn in a bowl of three percent hydrogen peroxide for about an hour. The peroxide will speed the healing process and relieve some of the pain.

Egg White

"My husband burned his arm on hot charcoal while emptying our hibachi grill. He was in severe pain. His arm had already turned bright red and was starting to swell. I remembered my grandmother's burn cure and took an egg out of the refrigerator, cracked it open, and smeared the burn with the white of the egg. After five minutes, the pain was completely gone. After the egg dried, my husband left it on his arm for about an hour. By morning his skin color had returned to normal with no blisters or peeling." — H.A.M., New Jersey, as reported in *Natural Home Remedies*.

Yogurt

Apply plain yogurt directly on the burn. After allowing it to dry, wash it off and reapply two or three more times.

Raw Chicken Fat

"A French-Swiss woman tried to lift a heavy pot of boiling water from the fire and, in doing so, slipped. She sustained scalds and second- and third-degree burns over a considerable area of her body, including the neck and chest. According to the doctor, her life was in danger. Fortunately, her husband ... got some fresh chicken fat and proceeded to spread it liberally over the parts of the body that had been scalded. Before long, the burning pain was relieved and his wife calmed down.... Within a few days the pain had completely gone and new skin was beginning to form over the scalded areas." — Dr. H.C.A. Vogel, in *The Nature Doctor*.

St. John's Wort Oil

Spreading St. John's wort oil over the burn helps relieve the pain and speeds the healing process. Also, helps prevent any blood poisoning that the burn may cause.

A Final Note

If a burn does not begin to heal within three to five days, or if it shows any sign of infection or becomes hot again, see a doctor immediately.

[*Many skin ailments can be healed by the simple application of colored light. Dr. William Campbell Douglass, author of* Color Me Healthy, *says that many skin conditions and burns can be helped, if not cured, with color therapy. According to Douglass, "This little-known therapy is an effective healer that's been used for almost two hundred years all around the world. I've read the results of thousands of cases. And I have seen many incredible successes." If you would like to learn more about color therapy and try the treatment for yourself, call 800-728-2288 and order* Color Me Healthy. *The price is $39.95 (which includes the treatment), plus shipping and handling, and it's worth every penny.*]

Chapter 23

Beating Colds and the Flu

Most of us are aware of the widespread range of the influenza virus (it strikes 10-20 percent of Americans each year), but few people are aware that 15,000 to 40,000 deaths are caused each year by flu-related illnesses. This means that proper prevention and treatment are crucial to fight this illness.

Identifying the flu is not as easy as it may seem. Health officials claim that many people who think they may have the flu, probably have a cold with flu-like symptoms. That's an easy mistake to make, since flu symptoms include a persistent high fever, chills, body aches and general fatigue, headaches, weakness that may last for several weeks, and intense chest congestion — many of the same symptoms as a cold. However, a cold rarely causes chills, and the aches and fatigue are usually mild.

What Causes the Flu?

Drug companies have tried their best to come up with a product that actually cures the flu. Many of them treat flu *symptoms*, but none has successfully treated the

Dr. Janitor's Magic Elixir

I don't know that I'd call it news from the scientific community, but Joe Murray, senior writer for Cox Newspapers, has an elixir that's a "miracle cure" for the common cold.

During Murray's years with the *Lufkin Daily News* he "came upon a young man, ... who was the very picture of health, a condition quite remarkable at the time, for it was the flu season....

"He was our janitor — but from that day on, I would always think of him, reverently and respectfully, as Dr. Janitor.... So it was that he shared with me that day the secret of his good health — the secret formula for Dr. Janitor's Magic Elixir, passed down through his family, through the ages — folk medicine for what ails you.

"Use only as directed:

"Gather half a dozen pine needles fresh from the tree. Wash them, break them into pieces and boil them in a two-cup pot of water for 10 minutes.

"Add the juice of half a lemon, a tablespoon of honey and a proper measure of appropriate spirits.

"Different people are of different minds concerning that last ingredient. I prefer a splash of dark rum. But an ounce and a half of gin seems to work well, too, as does vodka or bourbon.

"What you end up with is a cup of pine tree tea — a hot, tangy elixir containing the magic potion known as turpentine, as derived from distilling the pine needles.

"Drink the stuff as hot as you can stand it. Let it go down nice and slow, soothing your throat along the way." Recommended dosage: four times a day. (*Atlanta Journal*, 2/1/95)

virus. That's because until recently, very little was known about the cause of influenza. In the last 10 years, though, scientists have found that the illness is probably due to a dysfunction in the immune system, or a suppressed immune system.

In some illnesses, like chicken pox, the immune system can build up defenses to fight the virus for the rest of your life. So once you've had it, you usually won't ever get it again.

Herbal Product Inhibits Flu Virus

"Sambucol, an herbal product that contains extracts of black elderberries (Sambucus nigra L.) and raspberries (Rubus idaeus L.) has been shown in test-tube studies to inhibit the ability of the influenza virus to replicate (multiply). To determine the relevance of this finding to humans, individuals suffering from the flu were given either Sambucol or a placebo, in a double-blind study. Treatment was begun within 24 hours of the onset of symptoms and was continued for six days. Ninety percent of the individuals receiving Sambucol became symptom-free within two to three days. In contrast, those in the placebo group did not recover for at least six days. No significant side effects occurred." Sambucol is available through J.B. Harris, Inc., 4324 Regency Drive, Glenview, Illinois 60025, 800-941-7747. The price is about $11 a bottle. (*Nutrition & Healing*, April 1995)

But cold and flu viruses are constantly changing their biochemical properties, making it virtually impossible for the body to build up immunity. You may have immunity to one type of flu virus, but your body may never see that particular strain again.

This means we must rely on the body's general defense system to protect ourselves. If for some reason (such as poor nutrition, stress, poor sleep patterns, or anxiety) the system is not functioning properly, these viruses can invade.

Diet

Because flu viruses can do their most damage when the immune system is depleted, they are also a good sign that we need to improve our overall health. This includes

---

Flu Prevention

"My mother told us this story years ago. In 1918 in Germany when the flu hit hard, people were dying everywhere. Then a bird was flying around and singing, 'Eat garlic and you will get well.' Those who ate garlic got well. It may not have been a little bird, but another lady told me the following story in 1986. During the same flu epidemic of 1918, some robbers were robbing the dead bodies. When they got caught and taken to court, the judge asked them, 'Why is it that you never got sick?' They said, 'We ate garlic.'" — *H.K., Utah*

a healthy diet, which is a must if you want to have a healthy immune system. Eating processed foods, sugar, and chemicals is not the way God intended you to nurture your body.

Eating sweet-tasting foods can inhibit your body's ability to fight off infection. Any type of sugar, *even from orange juice*, decreases your white blood cells' ability to destroy bacteria and viruses. You need the vitamin C, especially while suffering from the flu, but you don't need the sugar. So take supplements and eat foods high in vitamin C, with little or no sugar.

You should also drink large amounts of fluids. This is exactly what your doctor will tell you if you go see him when you have the flu. He will graciously charge you $60 for the advice. But the fluids you need to drink include more than just water. Water will keep you from getting dehydrated, but it won't provide your body with the essential nutrients it needs to fight the infection. Water is absolutely essential, but also drink plenty of diluted vegetable juices and broths.

When you're sick, your body is telling you that it needs a rest. Rest will allow it to rejuvenate and strengthen the immune system that has been beaten down by overexertion or stress. A rest from foods that are hard to digest for the first day or two of the illness can also help. Go on a mini-fast for 48 hours. But remember, your body still needs an abundance of nutrients, so make sure you drink plenty of water, vegetable juice, and broths during your fast. (Fasting is not usually recommended for children under the age of 17.)

One vegetable in particular is especially effective for treating viral infections. Cherie Calbom and Maureen Keane, authors of *Juicing for Life*, tell flu sufferers to "increase your consumption of cabbage, which stimulates the body to produce more antibodies to combat infections. In the test tube, cabbage actually kills viruses and bacteria."

Easing Sore Throat Pain

"Once in a while, some of us develop a sore throat that makes it painful to swallow. Needed: a bottle of Sloan's Liniment and a cotton swab.

"Dip the cotton swab into the liniment. Standing before a mirror, open mouth and apply carefully to back of throat on either side of the uvula toward the side and downward. If done properly there will be a tendency to gag so do not overdo. There should be great relief in 15 minutes or less. If needed, repeat in one hour....

"This remedy was discovered accidently by a friend of our family over 60 years ago. He developed a cough and sore throat and was using a standard remedy for it. During the night he awoke and his throat was much worse.

"Without turning on the light he made his way to the medicine cabinet, took out what he thought was his medicine and took a small swallow. As he was gasping for his breath, he turned on the light and was horrified to see that he held a bottle of Sloan's Liniment in his hand. Nevertheless, he finally settled down and went back to bed. It was dreadful experience, but the next morning the soreness in his throat had entirely disappeared!" — *C.H.F., Virginia*

Diet and Prevention

Helping your body strengthen its immune system is something that you should be doing all the time, not just when you're sick. Start protecting yourself now by increasing your consumption of the following:

Garlic

Research has shown that garlic has strong antiviral activities. In October 1992, a team of German scientists found that garlic contains allicin and another half-dozen sulphur-based chemicals. That helped the researchers explain why garlic anti-viral properties work on such a broad scale — there are so many active compounds that each is effective on a specific range of viruses and bacteria.

Dr. William Campbell Douglass, editor of *Second Opinion*, reported, "The researchers tested garlic's activity against a range of viruses, including herpes simplex, parainfluenza type 3, vaccinia virus, vesicular stomatitis virus, and human rhinovirus. Here's the key: '*Fresh garlic extract was virucidal to each of the viruses tested.*'

"That was a phenomenal finding. Garlic extract killed *all of the viruses tested* including herpes, *influenza*, and the common cold. Again, our grandmothers were right: when cold and flu season hits, it's a good idea to increase your intake of garlic.

"And remember, ... garlic works best *before* the virus or infection takes a strong hold. At the first signs, start increasing your garlic intake to the equivalent of one clove per day. It just may work better than vitamin C."

Treating Colic with Herbs?

"Thirty-three colicky babies, aged two to eight weeks, were given an herb tea formula whenever they had a colic incident — up to three times in a day. Their colic was eliminated in more than 50 percent of them, according to their parents. The herbs used were anti-spasmodics: chamomile, vervain, licorice, fennel, and balm-mint. This study was reported in a 1993 issue of the *Journal of Pediatrics.*" (*Women's Health Letter*, 2/94)

Blueberries and Black Currants

Regular ingestion of these fruits is highly recommended during flu season. They contain high concentrations of anthocyanins, nutrients that possess antiviral and antibacterial properties. They also contain large amounts of vitamin C and vitamin A (4 oz. of blueberries contains about 1.6 mg of pure vitamin A). Combining the two in a juice is an excellent way to get these necessary nutrients.

Mushrooms

The Japanese have found that shiitake mushrooms contain a substance called lentinan. This substance is especially effective at fighting the influenza virus.

Two other foods that should be eaten generously during flu season are ginger, which destroys the influenza virus, and onions, which have strong antiviral and antibacterial activities.

Supplements

Eating the right foods during flu season is very important. This includes foods high in vitamins A, C, and E, zinc, selenium, and beta carotene. If you aren't getting enough of these, taking the proper supplements is a must. The *Journal of the American Medical Association* published an article by Dr. Henry Beisel showing how these specific nutrients have a significant effect on the activity of the immune system. (*JAMA*, Jan. 1981; 53)

It's a good idea to take the following supplements during the flu season. The dosages of certain supplements should be increased, as noted, during bouts with the flu.

Vitamin A is a strong immune system stimulant. Take 10,000-25,000 IU daily, 5 days a week.

Vitamin C stimulates the immune system in several ways. It helps repair tissue damage, acts as an antioxidant, and is essential to the white blood cells' ability to fight disease. The easiest way to take vitamin C during a bout with the flu is to mix the powdered form into a glass of water or juice. Take 1,000 mg, 1-3 times daily; increase to 1,000 mg every few hours during illness. If this upsets your stomach or causes diarrhea, you can reduce this dosage.

Vitamin E is another antioxidant that stimulates the immune system and aids in fighting viruses. Take the dry form, 200-400 IU, 1-3 times daily.

Zinc helps the body absorb vitamin A and may have some antiviral properties. It also helps the immune system's natural killer cells function properly. When you're sick, zinc can be taken easily in the form of a lozenge that can be purchased at most health food stores. Limit the number of lozenges you take in a day to six. Take 15-50 mg, 1-3 times daily.

Selenium works to make vitamin E a more effective immune-system stimulant. Take 50-100 mcg, daily.

Beta carotene is a strong immune strengthener with essential antiviral properties. Take up to 15 mg, once daily.

In addition to these supplements, there is a widely used flu-fighting herb you might want to try. Echinacea is an immune-system stimulant that was used by the early settlers to treat colds and flu. It has achieved worldwide fame in the latter half of this century for its antiviral, antifungal, and antibacterial properties. It has even been used to treat AIDS.

Mix five milliliters (about two droppersful) of echinacea tincture or a combination tincture of echinacea and goldenseal with water or juice. Take this every three to four hours during the first couple of days of acute symptoms. Most tinctures sold at the health food stores are an alcohol extract, but if you are sensitive to alcohol, make sure you purchase an alcohol-free echinacea-goldenseal tincture.

Summer Colds and Chicken Soup

Few things seem more miserable or more frustrating than having to suffer through an untimely summer cold. Summer's the time of year when you want to feel good about life; run and play and enjoy the outdoors. Not sit at home with congestion and a sinus headache.

Well, if you're one of the unfortunate ones that gets hit by the cold bug this summer, make sure you eat plenty of chicken soup. I know that sounds like an echo from the past when your mother would say the same thing, but trust me, it's good advice.

For centuries, moms have been feeding their cold-suffering children hot chicken soup to cure their ailment. In our world of antibiotics and cold medicines, many have considered this advice to be nothing more than an old-wives' tales. But what *is* the truth about this tasty treatment? Is it "good medicine" to eat homemade chicken soup when the sniffling and sneezing begins?

The very fact that this remedy has stood the test of time should tell you something. After all, it's not very often that you hear of one particular food recommended over and over again for a specific malady. But now, scientists are actually finding that chicken soup can be an extremely beneficial treatment for colds.

Back in the 1970s, researchers found that hot liquids increased the flow of nasal secretions. I'm not sure why it took a scientific study to prove that, but they did one nonetheless. An increase in the flow of nasal secretions helps the body rid itself of toxins and reduces the penetration of viruses, including the cold virus.

But chicken soup is not just another hot liquid. According to the March 1995 issue of *Runner's World*, "Stephen Rennard, M.D., a lung expert at the University of Nebraska Medical Center in Omaha, found that extracts of chicken soup inhibited the ability of certain white blood cells to participate in the body's inflammatory response. For test subjects, this meant they literally breathed easier, because their airways were less irritated and they produced less phlegm. Dr. Rennard believes this effect may result from the hundreds of active compounds found in the vegetables contained in soup."

Now you know why your mother always recommended eating chicken soup when you're sick. So here's the hard part: Can you make homemade chicken soup as good as she could? Well, if you can't, here's a simple recipe that's about as easy as they come (not including Campbell's). It only takes about five minutes to prepare and is ready to eat in 35-40 minutes.

1 chicken breast, cut in half (with the skin left on)
3 cans (13 oz.) chicken broth
1 package (16 ozs.) frozen mixed vegetables
1/2 cup celery, chopped
1/2 onion, chopped
1/2 clove garlic, chopped (more if you can stand it)
2/3 cup cooked rice or orzo (rice-shaped pasta)

Place the chicken breast in a medium sauce-pan and pour the broth over the chicken breast. Place over medium-low heat, cover, and cook for 20-25 minutes until the chicken is tender.

Remove the chicken from the broth and let it cool enough to handle. Pull off the skin; then remove the meat from the bone and cut into chunks.

Sauté the celery, onion, and garlic. While you're doing this, bring the broth to a boil. Stir in the mixed vegetables, sauteed herbs, chicken, and rice. Cook for five to 10 minutes until cooked through, stirring occasionally.

Makes approximately four to six servings. Happy eating!

Chapter 24

Grannies' Remedies for What Ails Ya

I was rummaging through a little hole-in-the-wall antique store the other day and found a most intriguing book. It was called *Grannies' Remedies*, so naturally I had to buy it. The book is about Mai Thomas's grandmother (with a taste of wisdom from other grandmothers) who had no formal medical training, but "yet for miles around people had more faith in her treatment than in the conventional skill of the local doctor with his top hat, wooden stethoscope, and mysterious little black bag."

This delightful little book is a collection of the remedies, wisdom, and experience of a healer who "lived in a grey stone cottage in a village on the borders of England and Wales" around the turn of the century. You've probably heard how Europe is having great successes with alter- native medicines and much of their wisdom comes from the healers of yesteryear — like Grannie.

Admittedly, some of Grannie's wisdom was more tale than treatment, but enjoyable nonetheless. Take, for example, these pieces of cold-prevention advice: Grannie insisted upon "persistent attention to the following rules:

Valerian Root and Insomnia

Researchers are finding that valerian root is very effective for treating insomnia, as well as anxiety, fatigue, and an unbalanced nervous system.

A double-blind study was conducted with more than 125 patients to test the effectiveness of an extract of the valerian root on insomnia. The study showed that the herb "improved sleep quality; lessened the time required to achieve sleep; and left no hangover effect in the morning. Another study showed that the extract improved sleep quality, time required to achieve sleep, and reduced night awakenings in persons suffering from insomnia. Additionally, this study also showed valerian reduced morning sleepiness.

"In other studies, valerian was shown to provide direct antispasmodic action on the gastrointestinal tract and might be helpful in the treatment of viral gastro-enteritis or of irritable bowel syndrome. In one study, 74 patients with rotavirus enteritis were divided into three groups with one receiving dosages of valerian. Within 72 hours, diarrhea stopped in 74 percent of the patients receiving the valerian and temperatures returned to normal in 91 percent of the patients receiving the valerian.

As a mild sedative, valerian may be taken in the following dose about 30 to 45 minutes before sleep is expected: Valerian extract, standardized to contain 0.8 percent valerianic acids, 150 to 300 mg. In some people, morning sleepiness may result, so a lower dosage is recommended. Additionally, if the dosage is not effective for the user, those factors that might interrupt sleep patterns, such as caffeine and alcohol, should be eliminated." (*Health Media Communications*, 3/95)

Walk with the toes turned outward. Walk with the chin slightly above the horizontal line, as if looking at the top of a man's hat in front of you, or at the eaves or roof of a house. Walk a good deal with your hands behind you. Sit with the lower part of your spine pressed against the chair-back."

There were some remedies that Grannie and her patients found to be especially helpful. For instance, take her remedies for insomnia:

"Warm, easily digested food is the most valuable of all sleeping draughts. Mental work should always be stopped half-an-hour before retiring and some relaxation indulged in, such as a short walk, exercise, or a not too exciting book. A sedentary life and intense mental work should be countered by periods of active exercise. Over-fatigue is best treated by a tepid bath or sponging, and a long draught of water before going to bed. A teaspoonful of salt in a pint of hot water is also useful...."

Plan B for Insomnia

"Decades ago I discovered a method to deal with the occasional bout with insomnia. This method is the common B vitamin: 500 mg of niacin taken with water at bedtime. Except for the first few times taking it, I never experienced the commonly known 'niacin flush.' But not knowing what effect large doses of niacin might have on my system, I did not use this method more than once every other evening. For me it worked very well without any adverse effects." — T.K.S., *Maryland*

"A remedy for insomnia suited to almost everybody is eating onions. Common raw onions should be taken, but Spanish onions, stewed, will do. This is due to a peculiar essential oil in onions. This oil has great soporific powers. Eat two or three onions, and the effect is magical.

"Take onion soup or syrup of onions every night. Onion jelly is also very soothing. To make it, shred two or three good-sized onions in a little stock and stew till tender. Add a squeeze of fresh lemon to make the onions digestible for the most delicate stomach, then pour in enough hot water for the quantity and thickness of the soup. Boil 10 minutes. Season and add a small piece of butter.

"When awakened and unable to sleep easily again, get out of bed, beat and turn your pillow, shake the bed-clothes well, then throw the bed open and leave it to cool. Meanwhile, walk about awhile, then return to bed.

"If you don't want to get out of bed, lift up your bed-clothes, draw in fresh air, and let them fall, forcing it out again. Repeat 20 times.

"Old people examined to assess the causes of their longevity agreed on one thing — all went to bed early and rose early."

That's just one small example of some of Grannie's wisdom. All of it might not be for you, but maybe you can find one morsel to chew on that will help you sleep better at night.

Chapter 25

Bee Stings & Insect Bites

It's the middle of the summer and your picnic is going great, except for one thing: those pesky little insects seem to be more attracted to you than anyone else. You know the feeling. It's almost as if the pests had zeroed in on you.

To be perfectly honest, they may have.

If your diet is high in fruit sugar you may have a difficult time getting away from the mosquitoes and biting flies. Fruit sugar can make the blood smell sweet and attractive to these insects. So if you know ahead of time that your plans include outdoor activities, you might want to avoid large amounts of fruit sugar.

Insect bites are one of the most irritating quirks about summer. We've all experienced that itchy little welt on the back of our leg or hand and tried desperately not to scratch — usually to no avail. But there are several simple ways to deal with the itch of a mosquito bite and the pain of a bee sting. If you've been bitten or stung, or want to avoid being attacked in the first place, try some of these simple remedies:

Repellents

One of the best ways to repel mosquitoes and blackflies is to take a large dose of vitamin B_1. *The Dictionary of the Best Tips and Secrets for Better Health* says that when you do, "you will eliminate what your system cannot assimilate through perspiration. This gives your skin a particular odor which repels mosquitoes and blackflies. The technique works best in hot weather, and especially if you tend to perspire a lot. Experiment to find

---

Fumigating Bee Stings

"Here in the Northwest, yellow jackets get very aggressive in the fall. Loggers, wood cutters, hikers — anyone eating outside — can become their prey. If you're stung, the fastest thing to stop the pain is to put gasoline on the sting and rub it in. The quicker you are, the faster the hurt stops. When my husband works out in the fall he carries a small glass bottle of gas in his shirt pocket.

"I was stung by a honey bee on the eyelid. I ran to the house and used a cottonswab to rub gas on it. Of course, the fumes hurt my eye, so I flushed the eye out after the gas treatment. No swelling appeared and the next morning my eye looked a little dark under it, like a bruise, but I went about my business and my circulation took care of it. I have seen other people who have had stings on their face swell up like a basketball." — *D.L., Washington*

the dosage that suits you best. Start by doubling the manufacturer's recommended dosage before going hiking in the woods."

In his newsletter *Health & Healing*, Dr. Julian Whitaker added to the evidence favoring vitamin B_1: "In 1943, Ray Shannon from St. Paul reported on 10 dramatic cases of resistance to mosquitoes from taking vitamin B_1 by mouth. In one gentleman who was constantly ravaged by mosquitoes while trout fishing, the vitamin allowed him to return home without a single bite while his fishing companions were covered with welts.... In a separate study, Dr. Shannon demonstrated that in 35 cases of itching from a variety of causes, vitamin B_1 was effective at relieving the itching in 62 percent of cases, and improving it in another 20 percent."

Besides this vitamin, many herbs, including pennyroyal, eucalyptus, calendula, and lavender, can be used as insect repellents. Gaea and Shandor Weiss, authors of *Growing & Using Healing Herbs*, have a simple recipe for making a natural repellent. "Combine 1/4 ounce each of penny-royal, eucalyptus, calendula, and lavender with two cups of rubbing alcohol in a closed glass container.

Mosquito Repellent

"Here are two things I've found to work effectively in repelling mosquitoes: (1) For short-term protection, apply vanilla extract the same as you would normally apply store-bought repellents. (2) For longer-term protection, always be sure that you're not deficient in 'B' vitamins." — *L.H.*

Let the herbs infuse for seven days, shaking the mixture daily. Then, strain and discard the herbs and bottle the repellent with a label listing its ingredients and the date made."

The mixture provides a cool, soothing effect when applied and should be reapplied often, as its effectiveness does not last for long.

Dealing With the Itch

If you are bitten by mosquitoes, apply some witch hazel, cider vinegar, or rub the bite with a slice of lemon or crushed tomato leaves. These will help relieve the itching. Straight lemon juice or the juice of figs are effective as well. Avon's Skin-So-Soft is another good repellant for mosquitoes, ticks, and other pests (call 800-FOR-AVON for a distributor in your area).

Other remedies include local applications of natural antibiotics like green clay (available at most health food stores) or brown-rice vinegar. Annemarie Colbin, author of *Food and Healing*, maintains that in addition to these topical antibiotics, insect bites respond well to the elimination of sweet juices and fruits in your diet. The sugar not only attracts the insects, it also stimulates the bite.

The most unusual treatment we've found for these annoying welts and stings is urine. Understandably, it's not a particularly popular treatment, but according to Dr. Whitaker, it even works for jellyfish stings.

If you're stung by a wasp, rub the sting with garlic, onion, or the white part of a leek. A pinch of meat tenderizer mixed with a drop or two of water to form a paste also works well for bites and stings.

The honeybee, on the other hand, is the only bee that leaves its stinger in your skin. In addition to the stinger it also leaves a sack that releases poison into your body. This sack will release even more poison if you squeeze the area around the sting or try to remove the stinger with your fingers or tweezers.

To remove the stinger, scrape it with a knife blade or a clean fingernail until the stinger has been extracted. After removing the stinger apply the meat tenderizer paste to help relieve the pain and swelling. Applying pure unprocessed honey is also good for bee stings.

The Weiss' recommend applying the following lotion to bee stings and insect bites: "In a large bowl, combine two pints of rubbing alcohol with one ounce dried echinacea root, one ounce dried plantain leaves, 1/2 ounce yellow dock root, and one bulb of chopped or pressed, peeled garlic. Cover the bowl with a plate or plastic wrap and let the mixture stand in a dark place for one week, shaking it daily. Strain and pour the mixture into a dark or opaque bottle. Apply it as a wash and/or a small poultice, using a piece of cotton gauze."

During the summer, everyone can expect to receive a visit from these pesky little insects at one time or another. But taking a few simple precautions and having the right type of treatments handy can make your next outing an enjoyable one. We hope that you and your family have a delightful and insect-free summer.

Chapter 26

Canker Sores and Cold Sores

When it comes to health problems that are more nuisance than serious trouble, canker sores and cold sores have to be at the top of the list. Their presence isn't life threatening, but the aggravation they cause can drive you insane. And what's worse, next to the common cold, these mouth sores are the most prevalent malady we have in the United States. You are not alone in your misery.

Generally speaking, determining the difference between a canker sore and a cold sore is fairly easy: one (the canker sore) is like a small ulcer inside the mouth, the other is known as a fever blister on the lips. There can be times when it is difficult to tell the two apart. They can appear on similar parts of the mouth and can often be treated with similar remedies. But that doesn't mean they are caused by the same problem.

Both conditions are usually self-limiting in nature, meaning that each sore will go away without treatment once it has run its course. But if you've ever experienced the pain of a canker sore or the humiliation of a cold sore (who wants to be kissed by an erupting fever blister), waiting until it runs its course is the last thing you want to do. The sooner you get rid of this "thing," the happier you'll be.

So let's look at some remedies that don't just make the sores go away, but make them go away *fast*. Then we'll see what we can do to keep the sores away *permanently*.

Canker Sores

Nothing can be more frustrating than sitting down to one of your favorite meals and realizing that every bite of it is going to be agony. You do your best to keep the

---

A Simple Canker Sore Cure

"I read your material about various means of controlling canker sores, but I don't recall seeing anything about using acidophilus. I have been using it for 30 years and it has kept me canker-sore free. I usually take two capsules twice a day, as well as eating yogurt three or four times a week. If I feel a sore coming on, I simply increase the dosage to four or five capsules three or four times a day. One day is usually all it takes to keep the canker sore from developing, but I usually take the increased dose for two or three days, just in case. I have recommended acidophilus to many people, and to the best of my knowledge, it has never failed to do the job." — *J.B., Huachuca City, AZ*

food away from the painful side of your mouth, but there's no way to keep from irritating a canker sore.

Currently, there are several over-the-counter medications you can use to dull the pain of a canker sore. None of them, though, have the ability to shorten the life of the ulcer, as most are pain relievers, not cures.

Canker sores, while not serious in and of themselves, can be caused by a variety of more serious conditions including anxiety, other emotional stress, or allergies. Stress is the culprit that most doctors and nutritionists blame for the majority of canker sore cases because of its effect on the immune system. When the body is functioning normally, the immune system is usually able to suppress the virus that causes canker sores. But when the body is under a great deal of stress, the immune system must work harder to fight disease. It can become weakened as a result, allowing the canker sores to appear.

Will Vitamins Work?

While we can't always avoid stress in our lives, we can help boost our immune system during stressful times with the proper administration of vitamins. The vitamins that help reduce the active time of canker sores vary from person to person, but you might try some of the following:

If you can catch the canker sore in its early stages, large doses of B complex vitamins taken orally will sometimes abort the attack. But once the sore is established, it doesn't seem to help much. Lavon J. Dunne, author of the *Nutrition Almanac*, says, "The B complex helps in the general condition of the skin, tongue, and digestive system. A well-balanced diet that provides adequate amounts of these vitamins protects against the formation of canker sores."

Dunne also indicates that zinc, taken orally (50 mg) or by topical application, has prevented or shortened the duration of canker sores. This was confirmed by the following testimonial in *Natural Home Remedies*: "I have experienced the misery of mouth ulcers (canker sores) for 40 years and have tried every remedy recommended by scores of doctors.... What works best for me is zinc gluconate. More than a year ago, I decided to experiment with zinc, since it is an age-old ingredient of many pharmaceutical preparations for skin problems. Zinc gluconate was a natural selection, since it is already available in a grade suitable for oral consumption. I pulverize several tablets by using a teaspoon and a tablespoon as a mortar and pestle. I then dip a moistened cotton-tipped applicator into the zinc gluconate powder and apply it topically to the ulcer every three to four hours. Healing is usually complete in two to three days instead of the usual week or more."

Others who suffer from canker sores have found relief with vitamin E oil. One person told *Natural Home Remedies* that she "had very bad sores on my tongue, gums, and cheeks for months.... I went to 12 different doctors. They prescribed all kinds of drugs and mouthwashes, none of which helped for more than a few days.

"Finally, I remembered reading that vitamin E was sometimes good for healing sores, so I bought a bottle of liquid vitamin E. I took several drops in my food. I also applied it directly to the sores in my mouth. Within three days, I noticed my mouth was hurting a lot less, and within a month my problems were practically gone."

Food Is Important, Too

Dr. Earl Mindell, author of *Shaping Up with Vitamins*, recommends increasing your "intake of foods rich in folic acid, iron, niacin, and vitamin B$_{12}$.... When the sores are painful, it's wise to keep away from tobacco; salty, tart, or rough-textured foods; as well as acidic beverages." (Although, for the stoic soul, salt applied directly to the sore has been known to kill the ulcer.)

Another food that has had some success in treating canker sores is yogurt. One particular child had suffered for years from canker sores. Since trying plain yogurt as an experiment, the child has been free from the sores for over a year.

Food Allergy

Many people believe they grow out of childhood allergies just be-cause the problem seems to disappear. Many times, however, the allergy remains, but manifests itself in different ways. For instance, as a child you might suffer from recurrent earaches that are caused by an allergy. But as an adult, that same allergy might affect the gallbladder instead.

Such is the philosophy behind Dr. Jonathan Wright's method of treating canker sores describes in his *Guide to Healing with Nutrition*. One patient Dr. Wright treated had endured a canker sore problem most of her life and also suffered from a gallbladder problem. After finding out the patient had a family history of gallbladder problems, Dr. Wright told her to avoid eating eggs.

The patient was bewildered until the doctor explained: "Don't misunderstand me: Eggs are a very good food. I usually recommend them, except for those who are allergic. I know allergic gallbladder sounds strange. I thought so too when I first read a report by Dr. James C. Breneman (board of regents, American College of Allergists) about it. I thought I'd try it out, though, and was amazed. The overwhelming majority of persons with gallbladder problems are very allergic.... Egg allergy is almost always present, along with a varying list of allergies to other foods."

The patient's allergy test "showed a distinct allergy to eggs, wheat, oranges, pork, honey, and brewer's yeast. Once she dropped those items from her diet, along with all vitamin products containing brewer's yeast, her recurrent canker sores cleared up. She's not had one in the three years since then.

"Canker sores are one of the many common manifestations of food allergy. Following the lead of Dr. Breneman, I always make sure to check for allergy, and find it frequently.... I've had individuals tell me that canker sores cleared up when they cleaned up their diets and took general vitamin and mineral supplementation."

If you know your canker sores are the result of food allergies, the treatment is obvious: don't eat the foods to which you are allergic. But if you're still getting the sores, you might try an herb called myrrh. That's right, the herb mentioned in the Bible. A mixture (which can be purchased at most drugstores) of myrrh and an alcohol solution can be applied to the sore with a cotton tipped applicator. This potion, which is also effective on cold sores, relieves the pain and accelerates the healing process.

The Fruit Juice Connection

Some of the most unusual findings on mouth sores came from research done by Dr. George Meinig, author of *"NEW"trition*. Dr. Meinig attributes the cause of most of these sores to organic acid foods. When acid juices like orange, tomato, grapefruit, and pineapple are consumed in large quantities, and sometimes even in small quantities, the number of ulcers that develop increases dramatically.

He said, "During 47 years of dental practice, I treated several thousand of these oral mouth ulcerations. In that time, I rarely saw a patient with this affliction who wasn't drinking fruit juice or eating fruit, usually in large quantities. A few could be traced to the use of chocolate or nuts, but most seemed related to citric acid fruits.... Way back in 1940, Harold F. Hawkins, D.D.S., reported in his book *Applied Nutrition* that many individuals would not completely digest the organic acid of some or all of these fruits, and if not, they could develop the symptoms of skin rash, edema, and apthae stomatitis (one form of cold sore), because of the acidosis that resulted. He also stated that this digestive inability was quite common in individuals with very low amounts of stomach hydrochloric acid enzyme and in those who had a low thyroid activity (hypothyroid)."

If you drink large amounts of fruit juice, remember that one glass of juice represents about four or five pieces of the fruit. That's a lot of acid for your stomach to digest — actually, it's too much. If you have a severe problem with mouth ulcerations, cut back on the fruit juice you consume. It might be the cause of your problem.

More on Cold Sores

Cold sores are symptoms of the virus herpes simplex (not the venereal disease) and much has been written about these unsightly blemishes. Unfortunately, the volume of writings has produced relatively few effective remedies. Many experts, in fact, maintain that the best cure for a cold sore is time.

Once contracted, the herpes simplex tends to remain dormant until the body is weakened by a cold or the flu (thus the name "fever blister"), extended exposure to intense sunlight, or, like canker sores, times of stress. The virus is extremely contagious while the cold sores are active, especially in the early stages, and activities such as kissing and sharing eating utensils should be avoided.

If you know you're going to be out in the sun for a long period of time, make sure you take along some sunscreen. When sunscreens with a protection factor of 15 or greater are applied on and around the lips, the development of cold sores is drastically reduced.

Simple But Effective

The simplest form of treatment that works for a few people is the application of ice to a freshly erupted cold sore. One physician that *Natural Home Remedies* mentioned said "he frequently suffered from painful cold sores that responded only slowly to every medical treatment he knew of, but invariably dried up in a day or two after a long kissing session with an ice cube."

A "long kissing session" simply means to hold the ice on the sore for at least 45 minutes. Some physicians have recommend "kissing sessions" as long as two hours, while others say that two to three minutes at a time, four times a day, for two days, works just as well. This is a harmless treatment, so experiment and use whatever works best.

Another handy remedy that can be purchased at any local drug-store is a styptic pencil. You're probably aware of its ability to stop the bleeding of cuts, but some people swear by its ability to stop cold sores. One gentleman told *Alternatives* newsletter, "If done at the first sign of a sore, only one application is needed. Used three or four times on a fully developed sore, it takes the pain away in one day, and the sore heals in three days with further applications once or twice a day."

Help from a Food Preservative

In addition, Dr. David Williams, the editor of *Alternatives*, says the food preservative Butylated Hydroxytoluene (BHT) is effective in fighting the herpes simplex virus. "Although herpes is generally thought to be incurable, there are thousands who have used BHT to eliminate its symptoms. The standard dose used with herpes is 250 mg daily, taken with the meal which has the highest fat content (BHT is fat soluble). Reports are that herpes lesions will begin to disappear within four or five days. If someone has difficulty digesting fats, it's possible the dose might have to be doubled (500 mg daily) until the lesions go away.

"After the herpes lesions have healed one should continue on 250 mg of BHT for a period of two weeks. After that time the BHT can be discontinued until another outbreak appears. Or 250 mg can be used daily as a maintenance dose to prevent future problems."

There is one particular side effect that you need to be aware of if you take BHT. It temporarily interferes with the liver's ability to metabolize alcohol. That means that if you drink spirits and take BHT, you could become intoxicated much sooner than normal. Also, anyone taking prescription drugs should consult their physician before taking BHT. And pregnant women, nursing mothers, and infants should not take BHT. No ill-effects have been documented, but this is not the time to experiment with a new synthetic compound.

BHT capsules of 250 mg can be purchased in most health food stores and are sold under the Twin Labs label.

How About Vitamins?

As we said earlier, many of the same treatments that work for canker sores are also effective on cold sores. Take for instance vitamin E oil. Dr. Don Nead of Redding, California, after drying the sore, places 20,000 IU of vitamin E oil on a piece of gauze and applies it to the sore for 15 minutes. The *New Encyclopedia of Common Diseases* says that Dr. Nead's method "has reduced or eliminated the sore's pain in less than eight hours and, in many cases, healed the sore itself in 12 to 24 hours."

For larger, more severe sores, the treatment can be increased to three times a day for three days. Dr. Nead claims that he has had a 100 percent success rate with vitamin E.

Or Lysine?

Lysine is an amino acid that has caught the attention of researchers trying to find a cure for the herpes simplex virus. While lysine is not yet considered a cure, Dr. Christopher Kagan of Cedars-Sinai Medical Center in Los Angeles observed that lysine counteracts the amino acid arginine, a known promoter of the reproduction of herpes. In addition, his research discovered that lysine supplements will also suppress the virus.

What does that mean to you? Two things: first, it means that if you have cold sores on a regular basis you need to avoid any foods that are arginine-rich. A mere two ounces of peanuts or chocolate have enough arginine in them to cause severe herpes outbreaks. Gelatin (Jell-O) is another food that should be avoided.

Second, according to the *New Encyclopedia of Common Diseases*, Dr. Kagan's research indicates that taking 800 to 1,000 mg of L-lysine daily caused the pain of cold sores to disappear overnight "in every instance." The supplement also prevented the development of new sores and healed the sores much faster than normal. Most physicians recommend taking two or three L-lysine capsules of 500 mg each, three times daily.

But even more importantly, Dr. Kagan's team of researchers found that lysine helped reduce the "frequency of recurrences. Patients who sought help because of the persistence and frequency of infection were maintained infection-free while on lysine."

Lysine's biggest drawback is its price. It tends to be quite a bit more expensive than most vitamins, but if you have recurring cold sores, it could be worth the price. It can be purchased at most health food stores. Make sure you buy the supplement called L-lysine. The plain form of the amino acid called lysine is not effective.

Many cases of canker sores and cold sores can be very difficult to cure. But with some simple experimentation and a little detective work, most will eventually yield to one cure or form of prevention. Most importantly, be patient. Many of these remedies are very effective, but the cure may not always be immediate.

Chapter 27

Questions and Answers

Canker Sores

Q. In addition to the treatments you've already mentioned, are there any natural treatments for canker sores? My oldest son gets them all the time and I always wonder if there's something wrong with him.

A. Several Scottish researchers undertook an extensive six-year study with 330 patients that indicated poor nutrition was a major cause of canker sores. As reported in the *New Encyclopedia of Common Diseases*: "Nutritional deficiencies were discovered in 47 patients, or 14 percent of the group. Of those 47, 23 were deficient in iron, seven in folate, six in B_{12}, and 11 suffered combined deficiencies."

The deficient patients were treated with the necessary iron and vitamin supplementation and the results were striking. All of the patients had suffered from "recurrent bouts of canker sores throughout their lives, but 23 were completely healed, meaning that they were free of canker sores for at least six months after receiving the supplements. In 11 others, there was definite improvement, with the ulcers appearing only occasionally. According to the researchers, the patients' prompt response to supplement suggests that the nutrients may directly affect the mucous lining of the mouth where canker sores occur."

A word of caution: Don't begin a regimen of iron supplementation before having your iron levels checked. Too much iron can cause some serious problems, so check with your doctor before you start.

Sunburn

Q. Fair skin runs in my family and, as a result, we all have trouble spending very much time in the sun. Are there any alternatives to the sunblocks we usually buy from the store? We've heard rumors that these may cause cancer.

A. Because 20th century man spends so much time inside under artificial light, our skin is no longer accustomed to spending lengthy amounts of time outside. When we go to the beach after a long winter, our skin is not prepared to handle the intense rays of the sun for a long period of time. That's why we get burned. And those with naturally pale skin are even more susceptible.

To combat the problem, our culture spends millions of dollars on synthetic lotions, whose safety is now being questioned. In his book *"NEW"trition*, Dr. George Meinig says there is a better way to help our skin acclimate to the summer sun. Para Amino Benzoic Acid (PABA) is a vitamin of the B complex family that can be of great benefit. "When taking a 100 mg. tablet of PABA one to three times per day, many can tolerate 50 to 100 times more sun than before. Red-haired people have particularly sensitive skin. I can report one red-headed lifeguard who now has comfortable summers because he uses PABA tablets and ointment....

"I would buy straight PABA ointment when possible. Many people prone to skin cancers find this regime stops the appearance of new sores and at times arrests their growth."

Don't get carried away with PABA, though. It's not a miracle drug that will allow you to spend endless hours in the sun with no recourse. You can still get burned, so limit your exposure time at the beginning. This will allow your skin to "warm up" to the sun. PABA can be purchased at most health food stores.

Eczema

Q. My doctor says that the redness, itching, small blisters, and the discharge of fluid from my skin is a disease called eczema. Are there any natural remedies for this type of skin ailment?

A. There are many skin diseases that have similar symptoms to those associated with eczema, but do not share the same cause. However, most of these disorders will respond to proper vitamin and mineral supplementation. In addition to avoiding dairy products, Dr. Jonathan Wright indicates in his *Book of Nutritional Therapy* that eczema patients should take the following supplements until the condition clears up:
1. **Zinc:** 50 milligrams, chelated, three tablets daily.
2. **Vitamin C:** 1,000 milligrams, twice daily.
3. **Cod-liver oil:** one tablespoon daily.

4. **Vegetable oil (soy, safflower, sunflower, etc.):** one tablespoon daily.

5. **Pancreatic enzymes:** two tablets with each meal.

Dr. Wright goes on to say that zinc and vitamin C are the most important nutrients for proper treatment of eczema. "In fact," he says, "the majority of cases of atopic dermatitis will get better with zinc and vitamin C alone." Try this first.

It will probably take at least two weeks before any improvement is noticed and, in extreme cases, it could take several months for the problem to clear up. Once it has cleared up, cut the zinc intake in half, and begin eating a little ice cream. If your skin stays clear, you can try experimenting with other dairy products.

Poor Eyesight

Q. I am 46, nearsighted, and have noticed that my eyes are getting worse. Is there a vitamin I can take or something I can do to help see better?

A. To see just how extensively poor eyesight is affecting our society, take a trip to your local shopping mall and notice the number of eye-care centers that are popping up. You can hardly get through the mall without seeing two or three new stores. So your problem is not unique.

The massive number of people needing eyeglasses for nearsightedness can be attributed to several factors. Researchers have found that in many cases the degree of nearsightedness is directly proportional to the amount of refined carbohydrates in the diet. Processed foods and sugar can also contribute to vision problems. And diets that are low in vitamin A (or low in zinc, which allow the proper release and metabolism of vitamin A) have been known to be a factor in night blindness.

Dr. Earl Mindell, author of *Shaping Up With Vitamins*, indicates that vitamin A "is the most important vision vitamin. It's necessary for clearness of eye tissues, especially the cornea or front surface of the eye. It prevents eye ulcers and is needed for the production of rhodopsin, a substance that allows us to 'recover' our vision after our eyes have been exposed to bright lights." Dr. Mindell recommends taking the following test to see if your body is vitamin A deficient: "Stare at a bright light for about 10 seconds. Then try to read something in large type. If it takes you more than a minute to see

Killing Fungus and Boils

"I have discovered two remedies that I use and find working 100 percent:

"1. I've had a fungus infection between the right foot two small toes for about 15 years. I consulted many dermatologists and used practically all pre-scribed and other preparations to no avail. Then I tried inserting a piece of Kleenex tissue between the toes daily. The fungus activity disappeared within 24 hours. I tried cotton and it doesn't work....

"2. Recently, I had a big boil ... and my doctor prescribed a full dose of antibiotic pills. Instead of using the pills, I started applying isopropyl rubbing alcohol on it twice a day. It was cured completely in about two weeks." — Z.Y., *California*

again, you might have a vitamin-A deficiency. (Dry, inflamed, or light-sensitive eyes can also indicate a vitamin-A deficiency.) Recommended supplement: 10,000-25,000 IU daily (for adults), five days a week."

The following testimonial from *Natural Home Remedies* shows the real value of vitamin A: "Some time ago I began having trouble with my eyes. I noticed the light was too bright when I opened the drapes in the morning. It made my eyes water. Then my glasses didn't seem to be right for me anymore. I couldn't see well enough to read very well. I thought I needed to have them changed....

"I didn't know what to do. Then I remembered reading an article about vitamin A being good for the eyes. I decided to try it as I had nothing to lose. I was taking 10,000 units at the time, so I took 25,000 units more. It was almost like a miracle! Within a week I found that my glasses were okay. I could see as well as I used to, and the light no longer bothered my eyes...."

If you notice that your eyesight continues to deteriorate after trying a vitamin A supplementation, you might consider getting contact lenses. Many times contacts will completely stop the deterioration of your vision.

Psoriasis

Q. My son has been suffering with psoriasis for six years and the doctors have not been very successful in helping him. Is there anything we can be doing at home to help this problem, or at least relieve the discomfort?

More on Boils

"This remedy was given to my mother by a barber ... back in the early 1930s. I was a young boy at the time and our barber noticed that I had several boils on my neck. My mother told him that I had them occurring off and on all over my body. They were very painful, especially when I had them lanced. The barber said that he had the same problem until this remedy was passed on to him....

"The remedy, he told me, was [to drink] about 1/4 of a flat teaspoon full of black gunpowder mixed in apple cider. It could be mixed in most anything, but apple cider has such a strong taste that it would mask almost anything that was mixed in it. I took the remedy ... and the boils slowly began to disappear. I have never had a recurrence to this day. My brother had the same problem, one shot and he too had a lifetime cure....

"Now, I am not naive enough to think that it was the explosive qualities of the black gunpowder that cured the problem. It must have been one of the chemicals in the substance that produced the miraculous effects. Black gunpowder consists of charcoal, sulfur, and potassium nitrate (sometimes sodium nitrate instead of potassium nitrate). I doubt very much that the tiny amounts of charcoal or sulfur that I took had anything to do with it, since we get small amounts of these chemicals in the food we eat. So, it must be the potassium nitrate that was doing it." — *G.L.H., California*

A. "The heartbreak of psoriasis," as the TV commercials used to call it, is an accurate description of a disease that is synonymous with misery for those it afflicts. Psoriasis is a skin ailment that is usually characterized by red patches covered with light silvery scales. The skin underneath the scales is thickened from inflammation.

Unfortunately, psoriasis has a history of being a very difficult disease to heal and is considered incurable by most orthodox doctors. But now, thanks to some not-so-orthodox research, there exists "intriguing evidence that fish oils may help prevent and relieve the symptoms of psoriasis."

This evidence, as cited by Jean Carper in her book, *Food: Your Miracle Medicine*, was the result of a British study conducted by researchers at Royal Hallamshire Hospital in Sheffield. The study revealed "that a dose of fish oil, equal to eating five ounces a day of an oily fish such as mackerel, 'significantly' alleviated symptoms, particularly itching, within eight weeks."

Another study "found that 60 percent of a small group of patients had mild to moderate improvement — less redness and itching — after eight weeks of taking fish-oil capsules. Other studies, however, have not found much, if any, improvement from fish oil.

"Still, since psoriasis is an inflammatory disorder, and fish oil is an anti-inflammatory, it makes eminent sense to eat more oily fish. Over time, such tiny infusions of the oil may do some good. The part of fish oil most effective is eicosapentaenoic acid (EPA), which is particularly concentrated in salmon and mackerel."

Carper added that it would be wise to cut back on other pro-inflammatory foods like animal fats, corn oil, sunflower oil, safflower oils, and any margarines or shortenings made from these oils. Fish oil supplements can be purchased at most health food stores.

Shingles

Q. Do you have any remedies for shingle pain? I've looked everywhere, but have found nothing that works. Since I have occasion to be concerned about this, I'm really needing something that can give me relief.

A. Sometimes the best remedies don't come from doctors, but from patients. The following remedy comes from the "Health Hints From Readers" section of *Alternatives* newsletter. Paul R.M. of Portsmouth, Ohio writes: "I want to share something with you that will be of significant relief to those who suffer from shingles.

Help for Shingles

"In 1959, my mother came down with shingles in Northern Germany. She had a severe case and the doctors said she should have cotton undergarments for relief. She suffered two years with this painful disease. Several years ago, I had it, but because I was taking 400 units of vitamin E a day and a friend said, "Open the capsules and put the liquid on the rash," which I did — it cleared up almost overnight. We have since seen somewhat similar results on an older man here in Sebastopol." — *G.M., Sebastopol*

An Almost Sure Cure for Hiccups

"I happen to own a record of 10 straight days of hiccups. I don't mean a 15-minute spell and stopping. I mean 24 hours of continuous hiccups for 10 consecutive days. I lost weight, my heart started skipping beats, and I was so run down, I could hardly walk.

"For 10 days, my doctor tried every remedy in the book. Finally, he said, 'I'm going to try something different and see what happens.' He gave me this liquid and in about two minutes they stopped. Don't get me wrong, they didn't stop for life, but when they return, I'm ready. The name of the cure is 'Gaviscon.' This antacid comes in tablets or liquid.

"My aunt's brother-in-law had open heart surgery about a year after I had my hiccups. One night, just before midnight, I received a phone call and it was my aunt. She said, Bud, what was the name of that stuff you took to cure your hiccups.... She explained that her brother-in-law had developed hiccups and was in severe discomfort. The doctors couldn't get them stopped.

"I told her 'Gaviscon' and called her the next night to see what happened. She said the doctors were amazed, because they didn't know of this simple cure. His hiccups stopped within five minutes.

"All I have left to say is, since this happened to me, I have given lots of people my cure for hiccups and it has helped them all." — *H.B., Ohio*

"A brother-in-law of mine has had the most horrible case of shingles for the past five years. He tried everything, including the most expensive prescriptions, and nothing worked. He could not even wear a shirt without extreme pain.

"An old farmer friend of mine just got over a similar case of shingles. What did the trick was Sloan's Liniment. Just apply it to the affected areas with a ball of cotton.

"My brother-in-law tried it and he is a new man. It's the first help he's had in all these years."

Sloan's Liniment is an over-the-counter product that can be purchased or ordered from most drug stores or pharmacies.

Sweaty Hands

Q. I have a question regarding my daughter, who is now 16. For a number of years, since she was about 8 or younger, she noticed her hands and feet would sweat for no reason. They have been cold, sweaty, clammy, etc. and it bothers her, especially now that she is a teenager. We have done everything possible and it has been diagnosed as overactive sweat glands. Can you recommend anything? We are willing to try anything that you can advise us on. She would be forever grateful.

A. When you're a teenager, the smallest of maladies (a pimple, for instance) can be a monumental blow to your self-confidence. And having a problem like excessively sweaty palms is no different — if not worse. Fortunately, there are some things you can do to deal with this occasional but frustrating problem.

Prevention magazine recommends using tea bags. "Hold a wet tea bag in your palm for 10 to 15 minutes each day. You may need to do the treatment for one to three weeks before the big event, suggests Karen Burke, MD, PhD, dermatologist and research clinical member at Scripps Clinic and Research Foundation in California. The tannin in tea (regular tea — not herbal) is an astringent. Its ability to shrink pores may create a comfortable decrease in sweat."

Dr. Burke also says that witch hazel or alcohol wipes will usually give temporary relief. "These astringents shrink pores a bit and help diminish sweating," explains Dr. Burke. "Try rubbing medical alcohol wipes over your palms moments before you have to greet that new client."

More Cures for the Hiccups

"I've got a no-fail and simple cure for hiccups. It is a spoonful of pineapple juice. I have never seen it fail — even with tiny infants where a few drops is sufficient." — *R.L.B., New York*

"I offer you the following method for curing the hiccups that I have used many times and given to others (to my knowledge, it has never failed to get rid of them): Simply eat three red cherries — one right after the other. That's it! Try it the next time you get the hiccups — works every time." — *M.D.C., Ph.D., Georgia*

And finally, you might try an antiperspirant. "The same stuff that keeps your underarms dry can work on your palms," says Dr. Burke. "Of course, you'll want to give this a test run before you try it on the public — you may be less comfortable with the feel of the antiperspirant than with the feel of the sweat itself."

Plantar Warts

Q. My daughter is 10 years old. She has three plantar warts on the bottom of her foot and nothing seems to work. Do you have any ideas?

A. The best medicine, by far, for warts of any kind is vitamin E. Taking it internally (200-1,200 IU daily) is said to work well, but the most effective mode of treatment is to apply the oil directly on the warts twice a day. Simply pierce a capsule and squeeze the oil onto the gauze pad of an adhesive bandage. Place the gauze pad over the wart in the morning and leave it on all day. Apply a fresh bandage with fresh oil before bedtime. It is best to wear a sock over the bandages to keep them from being knocked off.

You can also take 40,000 units of vitamin A internally daily plus three tablets of 6X Silicea three times daily. This is especially good for plantar warts, but scale back to 24,000 units after the warts disappear.

Scleroderma

Q. Our grown daughter has been diagnosed with scleroderma. She has a spot on her back that started by

looking like a spider bite, but spread larger and discolored like a bruise. Now it is about 2 1/2 inches in diameter, and is an almost round brown patch. It has become hard like leather. Do you have anything that can help her?

A. Scleroderma is an autoimmune disease that is marked by fibrous connective tissue in the skin and often in internal organs. This fibrous connective tissue can affect people in different ways. It has been known to make swallowing difficult by leaving the esophagus stiff and inflexible. When this happens, the food is not propelled down to the stomach as normal.

When treating scleroderma, the goal is to reduce the level of circulating immune complexes. Immune complexes are believed to contribute to the disease process by triggering the immune system against the body itself. This process eventually leads to harmful tissue damage.

Modern medicine treats scleroderma with corticosteroids, but there are natural supplements that are effective in relieving many of this disease's symptoms. Pancreatin, an enzyme from fresh hog pancreas, and bromelain, the protein-digesting enzyme of pineapple, are two preparations that have successfully reduced the level of circulating immune complexes.

Michael T. Murray, author of *Natural Alternatives to Over-the-Counter and Prescription Drugs*, reports, "Most studies have utilized the formulas marketed under the names Wobenzyme and Mulsal. However, it must be pointed out that these preparations are relatively weak in potency when compared with a number of enzyme preparations available in the United States. Presumably, by using higher-potency products, the impressive results demonstrated by Wobenzyme and Mulsal can be improved upon. It is preferable to use a full-strength undiluted pancreatic extract (eight to 10 times United States Pharmacopeia). Lower-potency pancreatin products are often diluted with salt, lactose, or galactose to achieve desired strength (e.g., four times or one time).... The dosage recommendation for 10-times pancreatin is 500 to 1,000 milligrams three times a day, 10 to 20 minutes before meals.

"The standard dosage of bromelain is based on its m.c.u. (milk clotting unit) activity. The most beneficial range of activity appears to be 1,800 to 2,000 m.c.u. The dosage for this range would be 400 to 600 milligrams three times daily, on an empty stomach."

Murray also points out that these preparations should be taken in conjunction with beta carotene (50,000 IU), vitamin C (3-8 grams), vitamin E (800-1,200 IU), manganese (15 milligrams), selenium (200-400 micrograms), and zinc (30-45 milligrams) every day.

Splitting Fingernails

Q. I have vertical ridges on my nails that regularly split. Cutting and filing them so they don't catch on everything doesn't work. What's causing this? What can I do to correct it?

A. Dr. Jonathan Wright, author of *Healing with Nutrition*, has had substantial experience with patients with brittle fingernails. There are a number of reasons the nails become brittle, but Dr. Wright says there is one main cause:

"Poor quality fingernails are usually only one of a whole collection of symptoms caused by suboptimal diet and poor digestion and absorption in a large majority of people.

"Easily cracked, chipped, peeling, and breaking fingernails are a key symptom in nutritional medicine. More than 90 percent of the people with poor fingernails tested in our laboratory don't have enough stomach acid....

"Unfortunately, it's not unusual to have low (or no) stomach acid and no symptoms at all. Although the older we get, the more frequent stomach malfunction becomes, it's relatively common even among people in their 20's and 30's....

"The key items for fingernail improvement appear to be protein and calcium, neither of which is well digested or absorbed by individuals with hypochlorhydria. Other nutrients are important, too, as fingernails are made of more than just calcium and protein. In practice, however, these make the biggest difference.

"Recently, improvement in fingernail quality through the use of essential fatty acids, specifically those found in primrose oil, have been reported. I've not yet had very many occasions to recommend primrose oil specifically for fingernail improvement, since digestive correction, calcium, and protein usually suffice (and primrose oil is expensive), but the times it's been tried, it appears to have been helpful."

Dr. Wright recommends having a gastric analysis done to see if your stomach is producing enough acid. If it's not, he prescribes five grains of betaine hydrochloride per meal, building up to 45 grains per meal. Also, make sure you don't take aspirin or any anti-inflammatory drugs with the hydrochloride. And don't take the hydrochloride if it makes your stomach hurt.

Macular Degeneration

Q. About two years ago, I was diagnosed as having macular degeneration — dry type. I was told there is not much that can be done in the way of treatment. The doctor did suggest that I start taking minerals such as zinc, magnesium, etc. I've been taking these for the past six months (daily), along with vitamins B_6, C and E, selenium, and beta carotene. So far there has been no improvement, but the problem isn't getting any worse. Do you have anything that might improve my outlook?

A. Macular degeneration, a deterioration of the center of the retina, is the leading cause of blindness in persons over 65. The fact that your problem is not getting any worse is a big step in the right direction. As far as supplements are concerned, you're taking the ones most recommended for this condition — and it looks like they are working. But there may be at least one more thing you can do:

"According to a new study, some lesser known substances in our diet may be even more important for maintaining healthy eyes. These compounds are called carotenoids (carotene-like molecules). Although beta carotene is the best known among this class of nutrients, other carotenoids also have beneficial effects. Two specific carotenoids, lutein and zeaxanthin, found in dark green, leafy vegetables such as spinach and collard greens, appear to be especially helpful for the eyes."

The study was conducted by Johanna M. Seddon, associate professor of ophthalmology, Harvard Medical School and Harvard School of Public Health, and director, epidemiology unit, Massachusetts Eye and Ear Infirmary. In a group of 876 elderly individuals, Seddon found that "those who ate the largest amount (top 20 percentile) of foods that contain lutein and zeaxanthin had 56 percent fewer cases of macular degeneration, compared to persons who ate the least amount (bottom 20 percentile) of these foods.

Carrots and yellow vegetables, which are high in beta carotene, were also protective, but not nearly as much as the dark green vegetables." (*Journal of the American Medical Association*, 1994;272:1413-1420; *Nutrition & Healing*, 2/95)

Epsom Salts

Q. I pulled a muscle in my leg the other day and a dear friend told me that sitting in a hot, epsom-salt bath would help sooth the pain. It worked wonderfully! It also made me very curious — can epsom salts be used for anything else?

A. Actually, epsom salts can be used for a variety of treatments. The mineral crystal is best known for its soothing properties in foot baths. But the Epsom Salt Industry Council says that the inexpensive mineral salt also can be used in a number of quick-and-easy ways:

"■ *For smoother skin* — To cleanse and exfoliate skin, massage handfuls of Epsom salt over wet skin, starting with the feet and continuing up toward the face. Then, take a bath containing two cups of Epsom salt and warm

Infertility in Men

"One hundred men with infertility apparently caused by abnormally functioning sperm cells (poor motility) were given three grams per day of L-carnitine for four months. After L-carnitine therapy, there was a significant increase in the proportion of sperm cells that showed normal motility. The improvement was greatest in men whose pretreatment sperm motility was the most impaired....

"L-carnitine, a vitamin-like compound, is found naturally in food and is also manufactured in the body. The chief function of L-carnitine is to transport fatty acids into mitochondria where they are metabolized to produce energy. Because sperm cells require a great deal of energy to 'swim' to their destination, an adequate supply of L-carnitine is essential. Previous studies have shown that the L-carnitine content of semen is reduced in men with low sperm motility. Apparently, sperm cells cannot swim normally unless there is enough L-carnitine around."

L-carnitine can be purchased at most health food stores and is completely nontoxic. While it is relatively expensive, it may be worth a try for male infertility. Most experts recommend a daily intake of 300 mg. (*Andrologia*, 1994;26: 155-159; *Nutrition & Healing*, December 1994)

water. The natural action will soften skin while easing kinks and stiffness in muscles.

"■ *For oily hair* — Add three tablespoons of Epsom salt to a half-cup of liquid shampoo made for oily hair — Epsom salt soaks up excess oil from hair. Apply one tablespoon of this mixture to dry hair and massage well. Rinse with cold water. Next, add juice of one lemon to a cup of lukewarm water. Pour juice on hair and leave for 10 minutes. Finally, rinse well with cool water.

"■ *To dislodge blackheads* — Add one teaspoon of Epsom salt and three drops of iodine to a half-cup of boiling water. After the mixture has cooled a bit, dip strips of cotton into the solution and apply to the problem area. Repeat three or four times, reheating the solution if necessary. Then gently unclog pores, and go over the area with an alcohol-based astringent.

"■ *For hair spray and gel buildup* — Combine one gallon of distilled water, one cup of lemon juice (fresh bottle), and one cup of Epsom salt. Cap the mixture and let it sit. The next day, pour the mixture onto dry hair and let it sit for 20 minutes. Then shampoo as normal.

"■ *To add body to hair* — Combine three tablespoons of deep conditioner with three tablespoons of Epsom salt. Microwave the mixture for 20 seconds. Work the warm mixture through your hair from scalp to ends and leave on for 20 minutes. Rinse with warm water. Promotes body and life in hair and restores curl to permed hair." (*Let's Live*, 2/95)

Poor Night Vision

Q. Over the last couple of years, my wife's ability to drive at night has deteriorated severely. It's to the point now that I get real nervous when she has to drive in the dark. Is there anything she can take to help her situation?

A. Actually, there is an herb that has gained considerable popularity in the last few years for helping "night blindness" and eyesight in general. It's bilberry, and study after study has been reported in the European journals confirming the positive benefits of this herb on vision. Unfortunately, it hasn't received the attention it deserves in the United States.

"During World War II, Royal Air Force (RAF) pilots were forced to fly at night in order to accomplish any deep assault on Germany. Many pilots and their crew members complained of the poor visibility and its effects on their performance. Pilots noted that if they took bilberry jam, their night vision improved. Researchers found 50 years later what the RAF already knew, that bilberry's powerful effects increased retinal purple (rhodopsin) by dramatic amounts in just 20 minutes, sometimes less. One study showed bilberry to improve eyesight and increase ocular blood supply in 75 percent of patients. It improved nearsightedness after five months of regular use, while an 83 percent improvement in visual acuity was recorded after only 15 days. One of the more encouraging statistics regarding bilberry's visual enhancing properties is that over 80 percent of the people taking bilberry for the first time improved on their visual acuity exam and passed a night vision test. Long-term improvements took an average of six weeks with regular doses." (*Medical Herbalism*, Winter/94-95)

You can purchase bilberry in a commercially prepared extract or in capsule form at your local health

Infertile? Avoid Caffeine

"Women who are trying to conceive may want to limit caffeine consumption, according to a study funded by the National Institutes of Health (NIH).

"Researchers surveyed nearly 2,000 newly pregnant women and found that those who regularly drank 300 or more milligrams of caffeine daily (about three cups of coffee, nine cups of tea, or six cans of caffeinated soda) were 27 percent less likely to conceive during each menstrual cycle. Women who drank less than 300 milligrams of caffeine each day were 10 percent less likely to conceive each month. Overall, 90 percent of the women became pregnant within a year.

"According to Elizabeth E. Hatch, Ph.D., an NIH researcher who conducted the study while at the Yale University School of Medicine, more research is needed to determine whether caffeine or another substance in caffeinated beverages is the culprit." (*Parents*, 10/94)

food store. Of the capsules, take one capsule up to three times daily. Or mix 15 to 40 drops of the extract in water or juice and drink three times daily. While both forms are safe, be very cautious not to take more than the recommended dosage; bilberry leaves can be poisonous if consumed in excess over an extended period of time.

Alzheimer's Disease

Q. My wife is beginning to suffer from Alzheimer's disease. Is there anything we can do to prevent the disease from getting worse or to cure it?

A. Nothing in orthodox medicine today offers any help to the four million people who suffer from Alzheimer's.

However, Dr. David Williams, editor of *Alternatives for the Health Conscious Individual*, reports in his March 1994 issue that work is currently underway to start testing a new drug that has been used successfully on hundreds of patients in Shanghai. The drug, Huperzine A, is made from the active ingredients of a plant called club moss. The Chinese have used this plant for centuries to brew tea and they claim that drinking club moss tea improves memory and failing mental capacity.

While Huperzine A is not available in the United States, club moss (or Shen Jin Cao, as the Chinese call it) can be purchased in this country. However, it's not very easy to find unless you live near an area with a large Chinese population. If you can't locate the herb locally, there is a mail-order supplier who will sell it to health professionals, pharmacies, or health-food stores. Ask your doctor or health food store to contact Nuherbs Co. at 3820 Penniman Avenue, Oakland, CA 94619.

According to Dr. Williams, it's important to retain the medicinal properties of the herb when brewing the tea: "Use two teaspoons of dried herb per cup of boiling water. The dried herb should be placed inside a cup and then boiling water poured on top of it. Immediately cover the cup to prevent any medicinal components from being carried away with the steam. After the tea has set covered for three or four minutes, it can be strained into another cup for consumption. If desired it can be sweetened to taste with honey."

Hoarseness

Q. For my job, I am constantly giving boardroom presentations. Every now and then my voice gets

---

Yogurt and Yeast Infections

Women have been telling their doctors for years that eating yogurt has helped control their chronic vaginal yeast infections. But because these accounts were not supported by any scientific research, most doctors have refused to prescribe this simple treatment.

But now a study done at Long Island Jewish Medical Center has confirmed what women have known for a long time: "Eating eight ounces a day of yogurt containing live lactobacillus acidophilus cultures can prevent vaginal yeast infections."

Some women have also reported using the yogurt as a douche, instead of eating it. To date, no research has been conducted to prove the effectiveness of this method.

If you don't like yogurt or if you don't want to eat that much every day, you can purchase lactobacillus acidophilus in tablet form at your local health food store. (*Vogue*, 1/95)

hoarse, causing my presentations to suffer. Is there anything I can do to prevent my voice from going out on me?

A. If you watched Bill Clinton on television during the 1992 Presidential Campaign and into his first year of office, you remember seeing the effect that hoarseness can have on a person. Conventional medicine prescribed an antibiotic and rest for the president, but in the long run the antibiotics probably did more harm than good.

Next time your voice gets a little cracked, try one of these simple remedies from *The Nature Doctor*. Dr. H.C.A. Vogel suggests, "The berries of the mountain ash, also known as rowan, are a good remedy for hoarseness. There may be a tree in your garden, or in a neighbor's, or you may remember seeing one on country walks. At the same time, you can look out for the pimpernel. To combat hoarseness, chew either rowan berries or pimpernel root, fresh or dried. Keep chewing these for as long as possible and let the insalivated juice run down the throat. This simple treatment makes hoarseness disappear in no time at all. Of course, you do not need to use both remedies together, either one on its own will no doubt help you. When you have lost your voice, rowan berries and pimpernel root are two of the best cures available."

By the way, if you have a remedy for hoarseness, or any other ailment, let us know. We would love to hear about it.

Endometriosis

Q. I am a 25-year-old female who suffers horribly from endometriosis. Many times the pain is unbearable and the only solution my doctor can give is for me to get pregnant. Because I'm single that's really not an option. Is there anything I can do?

A. Endometriosis is a condition created when the endometrial tissue (the tissue which grows along the inside wall of the uterus and is shed each month with the menstrual cycle) grows outside the uterus around the fallopian tubes, on the ovaries, and across the ligaments that support the uterus. As it weaves its way through these internal tissues, the endometrial tissue can leave web-like scars. Then, during the menstrual cycle, it acts like normal tissue and swells and bleeds, only the discharge is stuck in the body. As a result, severe pain can be felt throughout the abdominal area from the inflammation and scarring.

Treating endometriosis is something that most doctors don't know very much about. They will usually tell you to get pregnant because it will usually cure, or at least help, the problem and because they don't have any other options. However, for single women this is not feasible and for one reason or another it may not be an option for many married women.

So what can you do? To start, avoid all foodstuffs that are connected with the reproductive system of animals or contain natural or artificial hormones. This includes milk and milk products, eggs, and the meat of animals raised on estrogen. Annemarie Colbin, the founder and director of the Natural Gourmet Cookery School in New York City and author of Food and Healing, says that this is the first treatment for problems related to the female reproductive system.

She said: "In my experience, such abstentions, coupled with a hearty health-supportive diet, have helped ameliorate symptoms in cases of ... endometriosis and infertility. Endometriosis is further helped by sexual abstinence during menstruation. It seems that coitus can push the secretions back up and through the fallopian tubes into the pelvic cavity. This endometrial tissue then remains there and causes acute pain and discomfort. Orthodox Jewish women, whose traditional customs keep them from having intercourse while they show the least bit of bleeding, have an extremely low incidence of endometriosis." She says that it usually takes from one month to 18 months for the conditions to reverse, depending on the severity of the problem.

Colds

Q. With winter just around the corner, I was wondering what kind of herb would be most effective in treating the common cold?

A. There are many herbs that can be used to treat the common cold, but let us bring to your attention a treatment that almost no one knows of anymore.

According to Dr. William Campbell Douglass, editor of *Second Opinion*, this herbal remedy was considered one of the most important by herbal experts. The herb is black mustard and is perhaps the best herb in the world for poultices.

Dr. Douglass states, "It is recommended that the poultice be applied *to the feet*, no matter what part of your body is crying for succor. Make a foot bath and add a tablespoonful or more of dried black mustard seed to the hot water. The theory is that the blood will flow away from areas of congestion and to the feet. This treatment works well for coughs, headaches, sinus congestion, and many other cold symptoms."

Black mustard seeds can be purchased at local nurseries and seed companies.

Earaches

Q. My 10-year-old son has suffered from earaches since he was an infant. His ears have always been blocked and are prone to infection. Attempts to drain his ears with plastic tubes have been unsuccessful. He can no longer go swimming because it guarantees the return of the earache and infection. The problem is starting to affect his hearing and is also causing him to fall behind in school. Is there anything we can do for him?

A. More than likely, your child's ear infection trouble is the result of a food allergy. Nutrition specialist Dr. Jonathan Wright wrote in his book, *Healing with Nutrition*, "The vast majority of children with recurrent earaches are allergic to food."

The food that is most often the cause of this food allergy is milk. In fact, says Dr. Wright, "milk is so usually a cause of recurrent infection in infants and small children that it's 'guilty until proven innocent.'" Wheat is another food that makes it on Dr. Wright's list of foods to avoid. But to be sure, you'll need the help of an allergist who uses the RAST blood test to identify allergies. The skin tests that most doctors use to determine allergies are useless in spotting a food allergy.

Prostate Problems

"As a man who has had for many years a continual bout with prostate problems, not major, but irritating nonetheless (diagnosis was always slight enlargement), I have tried several different "cures." I was on zinc pills for awhile, 50 mg daily (which helped), until a man suggested I try pumpkin seed oil capsules. I now take one pill of 1,000 mg daily. This has had a positive effect on nocturnal visits to the bathroom. A urologist laughed at me, saying 'how unscientific!' I replied, 'but it works.'" — *D.B., Arizona*

But there maybe other contributing factors involved in your child's problem. Refined sugar and processed foods significantly aid the growth of most infections. "Sugar," says Dr. Wright, "interferes with the ability of white blood cells to kill germs." And processed foods rob our body of the vitamins and minerals it desperately needs to stay healthy.

In addition to avoiding milk, sugar, and processed foods, there are several herbs that may help your child. The *Complete Medicinal Herbal*, by Penelope Ody, indicates that goldenseal in capsule form is a "powerful cooling astringent with a phlegm-reducing action. Take two 200 mg capsules ... three times a day." Other herbs that might prove beneficial include goldenrod (5 ml), purple coneflower (10 ml), and pasque flower (1-2 ml) in tincture form, taken three times per day.

Morning Sickness

Q. I've got an extremely weak stomach and the least little disturbance can make me feel nauseated, especially when I'm pregnant. Is there anything I can do to help the nausea? And all the better if it helps morning sickness."

A. You're not alone in this one. Just about everyone in the world experiences nausea sometime in their life — some more than others. There are a number of things that can cause nausea, from giving blood to credit card bills to reading in the car, and that's just to name a few.

One of nature's best medicines for nausea was recently discussed in Earl Mindell's *Joy of Health* newsletter (4/94). But Mindell didn't have to go to medical school to get this one. It was passed down to him by his mother.

Mindell writes:

"Ginger is a wonderful antinauseant, making it a safe remedy for morning sickness and motion sickness.

"When I was a little boy if I had an upset stomach, my mother always gave me all the ginger ale I wanted.

"What a clever woman. Ginger plus a high carbo-hydrate drink is a great antinauseant.

"Try one of these:

"Drink some gingerroot tea, chew a bit of fresh ginger, or take 1 to 2 ginger root capsules.

"Not too long ago an article in the *Wall Street Journal* lamented the fact that there was no drug for morning sickness after the drug bendectin was removed from the market. Fortunately, you don't need to wait for a 'new drug.' You can rely on a natural remedy that the Chinese used for centuries."

Tinnitus

Q. I've had tinnitus for five years or so and I was wondering if you have any alternative suggestions for dealing with this problem?

A. If you've ever fired a gun without any hearing protection, you know what it's like to have tinnitus. But people who suffer from this miserable problem have that ringing in their ears for prolonged periods of time. It can start out as a persistent little annoyance and gradually get to where it's an unbearable affliction.

There are many things that can cause tinnitus, everything from aspirin to hypoglycemia to a deficiency of a certain vitamin. If you suffer from arthritis and are taking aspirin to deal with the pain, you might try a different pain reliever. Aspirin, as well as many prescription drugs, can cause tinnitus and even deafness.

Some doctors believe that tinnitus is caused by hypoglycemia (low blood sugar). A diet high in refined carbohydrates causes the blood sugar level to drop, depriving the ear of the necessary nutrients, oxygen, and energy it needs to function properly. If you have symptoms of hypoglycemia, cut back on the refined carbohydrates and sugar and add a little more protein to your diet.

There are also well-documented findings that vitamin A supplementation may contribute to hearing improvement. Animal studies have found that the tissue in the inner ear has 10 times more vitamin A in it than any other tissue in the body. Deficiencies in other nutrients, including vitamin B_{12}, magnesium, chromium, and zinc, should also be checked.

Tinnitus can also be caused by toxins in the blood, so you might try fasting for a couple of days. If the ringing goes away while you're fasting, you have a pretty good indication that a toxin or food allergy is causing the problem.

Menorrhagia

Q. My daughter has had an excessive menstrual flow for quite some time, and nothing the doctors have tried works. They can't identify why she has it or how to slow it down. Can you please suggest something that will help this problem?

A. Excessive menstrual flow is one of the biggest problems in young women today. A woman can lose up to 92 percent of her total menses in the first three days. And while it gives the impression that your daughter is losing more blood than normal, she probably is not.

Menorrhagia is actually more of a symptom than an actual disease. It can be caused by vitamin and iron deficiencies, hypothyroidism, and abnormalities of the endometrium.

According to Dr. E. Cheraskin, "Two celebrated researchers looked at this problem in a group of presumably otherwise healthy young women. Each of the subjects in the experimental group received 600 mg of ascorbic acid/bioflavonoids (vitamin C) on a daily basis in dividend doses. The control patients were given an indistinguishable dummy pill. The results are clear.

Thirty-two out of 37 women displayed decreased blood loss when treated with the test capsules for two months, while only one in the control group improved." (*Health Journal*, Winter/95)

Bibliography

Alternative Medicine. Puyallup, Washington: Future
Medicine Publishing, 1993.

*Amazing Medicines the Drug Companies Don't Want You
to Discover*, Tempe, Arizona: University Medical
Research Publishers, 1993.

Balch, James F., M.D. and Phyllis A. Balch, C.N.C. *A
Prescription for Nutritional Healing*, Garden City
Park, New York. 1990.

Batmanghelidj, F., M.D. *Your Body's Many Cries for
Water*, Falls Church, Virginia: Global Health
Solutions, Inc. 1992.

Beverly, Cal, ed. *The Book of 1,001 Home Health
Remedies*, Peachtree City, Georgia: FC&A
Publishing. 1993.

Bricklin, Mark, William Gottlieb, Marian Wolbers, eds.
New Encyclopedia of Common Diseases, Emmaus,
Pennsylvania: Rodale Press. 1984.

Bricklin, Mark, *Natural Home Remedies*. Emmaus,
Pennsylvania: Rodale Press, 1982.

Calbom, Cherie and Maureen Keane. *Juicing for Life*, Garden City Park, New York: Avery Publishing Group, Inc. 1992.

Carper, Jean, *Food: Your Miracle Medicine*. New York, New York: HarperCollins Publishers, 1993.

Colbin, Annemarie. *Food and Healing*, New York: Ballantine Books. 1986.

Dehin, Robert, ed. *Dictionary of the Best Tips and Secrets for Better Health*, Chester, Connecticut: CCN Publishing, Inc. 1992.

Diamond, Harvey and Marilyn. *Fit for Life*, New York, New York: Warner Books, Inc. 1985.

Douglass, William Campbell, M.D. *Dangerous (Legal) Drugs*, Atlanta, Georgia: Second Opinion Publishing, Inc. 1994.

Douglass, William Campbell, M.D. *Hydrogen Peroxide: Medical Miracle*, Atlanta, Georgia: Second Opinion Publishing, Inc. 1996.

Duke, James A., *CRC Handbook of Medicinal Herbs*. Boca Raton, Florida: CRC Press, 1985.

Dunne, Lavon J. *Nutrition Almanac*, New York, New York: McGraw-Hill Publishing Co. 1990.

Gladstar, Rosemary. *Herbal Healing for Women*, New York, New York: Simon & Schuster. 1993.

Goodenough, Josephus, M.D. *Dr. Goodenough's Home Cures and Herbal Remedies*, New York, New York: Avenel Books. 1982.

Hausman, Patricia, Judith Benn Hurley. *The Healing Foods*, New York, New York: Dell Publishing. 1989.

Heinerman, John. *Heinerman's Encyclopedia of Fruits, Vegetables, and Herbs*, West Nyack, New York: Parker Publishing Co. 1988.

Heinerman, John. *Heinerman's Encyclopedia of Nuts, Berries, and Seeds*, West Nyack, New York: Parker Publishing Co. 1995.

Hylton, William H., Claire Kowalchik, eds. *Rodale's Illustrated Encyclopedia of Herbs*, Emmaus, Pennsylvania: Rodale Press. 1987.

Jensen, Dr. Bernard, *Foods That Heal*. Garden City Park, New York: Avery Publishing Group, 1993.

Kloss, Jethro. *Back to Eden*, Loma Linda, California: Back to Eden Books Publishing Co. 1939.

Kordel, Lelord, *Natural Folk Remedies*. New York, New York: G.P. Putnam's Sons. 1974.

Kowalchik, Claire, & William H. Hylton, ed. *Illustrated Encyclopedia of Herbs*. Emmaus, Pennsylvania: Rodale Press. 1987.

Meinig, George, D.D.S., F.A.C.D. *"NEW"trition*, Ojai, California: Bion Publishing. 1987.

Mindell, Earl, R.Ph., Ph.D. *Herb Bible*, New York, New York: Simon & Schuster/Fireside. 1992.

Murray, Dr. Michael T., *Natural Alternatives to Over-the-Counter and Prescription Drugs*. New York, New York: William Morrow and Company, 1994.

New Medicine Show, The. Mount Vernon, New York: Consumers Union. 1989.

Pahlow, Mannfried, *Healing Plants*. Hauppauge, New York: Barron's Educational Series, 1992.

Peason, Durk, and Sandy Shaw. *Life Extension*, New York, New York: Warner Books. 1982.

Petulengro, Gipsy. *Romany Remedies and Recipes*, New York, New York: E.P. Dutton & Co., Inc. 1936.

Skolnick, Susan A. *The I Feel Awful Cookbook*, Bethesda, Maryland: National Press, Inc. 1985

Thomas, Richard. *The Essiac Report*, Los Angeles, California: The Alternative Treatment Information Network. 1993.

Thomson, William A.R., M.D., *Herbs That Heal*. New York, New York: Charles Scribner's Sons, 1976.

Tkac, Debora. *The Doctors Book of Home Remedies*, Emmaus, Pennsylvania: Rodale Press. 1990.

Vogel, H.C.A, M.D. *The Nature Doctor*, New York, NY: Instant Improvement, Inc. 1993.

Walker, Morton, D.P.M. *The Chelation Answer*, Atlanta, Georgia: Second Opinion Publishing, Inc. 1994.

Weil, Andrew, M.D. *Natural Health, Natural Medicine*, Boston Massachusetts: Houghton Mifflin Co. 1990.

Weiss, Gaea and Shandor. *Growing & Using the Healing Herbs*, Emmaus, Pennsylvania: Rodale Press. 1985.

Wright, Jonathan V., M.D. *Dr. Wright's Guide to Healing with Nutrition*, New Canaan, Connecticut: Keats Publishing, Inc. 1988.

Index

S